INTRODUCTION TO VISION SCIENCE

Introduction To Vision Science

Richard A. Clement
Defence Research Agency,
Fort Halstead,
Sevenoaks,
Kent, U.K.

LAWRENCE ERLBAUM ASSOCIATES, PUBLISHERS
Hove (UK)   Hillsdale (USA)

Copyright © 1993 by Lawrence Erlbaum Associates Ltd.
All rights reserved. No part of this book may be reproduced in any form, by photostat,
microform, retrieval system, or any other means without the prior written permission
of the publisher.

Lawrence Erlbaum Associates Ltd., Publishers
27 Palmeira Mansions
Church Road
Hove
East Sussex, BN3 2FA
UK

British Library Cataloguing in Publication Data

Clement, Richard A.
  Introduction to Vision Science
  I. Title
  152.4

ISBN 0-86377-312-5

This book was produced from camera ready copy supplied by the author
Printed and bound by BPCC Wheatons Ltd., Exeter

To Christine, Blaise and Rosie

Contents

CHAPTER 1

Introduction

One of the most striking features of vision is that despite having two eyes, one is not usually aware of two separate images of the world. Rather one sees the world as though with a single conceptual eye, referred to as the CYCLOPEAN EYE, located midway between the two real eyes.

Hering (1879) introduced the idea of the cyclopean eye and provided a very simple but effective demonstration of how it works, which involves the following steps. First, stand at arm's length in front of a window and look out with the left eye only. Select a salient feature, such as a tree and make a mark on the window, at the position of the tree. Second, look out with the right eye only, in the direction of the mark and discern a distinct feature, such as a parked vehicle, in this direction. Finally, look with both eyes open, fixating the mark on window. What one sees is the tree and vehicle superimposed, demonstrating that the two lines of sight are merged into a common one originating at the cyclopean eye as shown in Fig. 1.1.

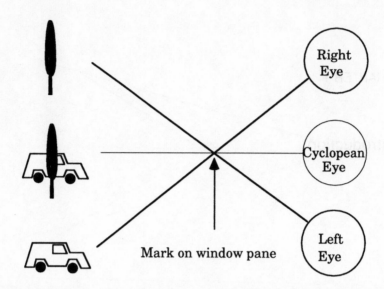

FIG. 1.1. Hering's window pane demonstration. When the left eye is aligned with a tree and the right eye is aligned with a vehicle, the two images are seen in the same direction from a cyclopean eye.

This cyclopean eye model explains the occurrence of double images that occur even with normal vision, a phenomenon known as PHYSIOLOGICAL DIPLOPIA. If two pencils are held upright and 100 millimetres apart along the straight ahead direction, then two types of diplopia can be distinguished. If the nearer pencil is fixated, as shown in Fig. 1.2, then the further pencil appears as a double image. In this and the subsequent figure, F denotes the point of fixation and P denotes the pencil which appears as a double image. Closing the left eye demonstrates that the image from the right eye appears on the right. Hence this type of physiological diplopia is referred to as UNCROSSED DIPLOPIA. If the further pencil is fixated, as shown in Fig. 1.3, then the nearer pencil appears as a double image. Closing the left eye demonstrates that the image from the right eye appears on the left. Hence this type of physiological diplopia is referred to as CROSSED DIPLOPIA.

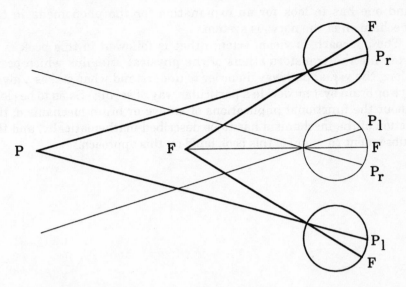

FIG. 1.2. Demonstration of uncrossed diplopia. F is the point of fixation and P_l and P_r are the images of the point P in the left and right eye respectively.

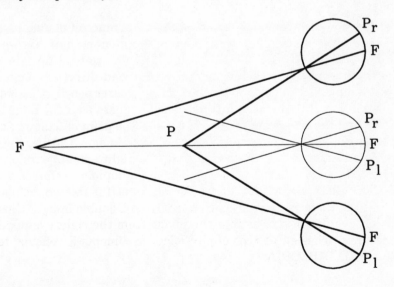

FIG. 1.3. Demonstration of crossed diplopia.

So what is the significance of the cyclopean eye? Obviously every object could be assigned a unique visual direction with respect to a point midway between the two eyes, but this is not what the brain does and one has to look for an explanation for the phenomena in the mechanism of the nervous system.

The approach to vision science that is followed in this book is to examine the transformations of the physical stimulus which occur along the visual pathway, in order to understand what makes a given eye or brain system decide a particular way of seeing. So as to be clear about the functional implications of an eye or brain mechanism, the action of the mechanism has to be described mathematically, and the subsequent chapters of this book build on this approach.

CHAPTER 2

Vector Algebra

The most difficult part of applying mathematics to the description of a physical phenomenon involves identifying the relevant aspects of the phenomenon. This is especially true of vision, as in any natural scene, it is not obvious what constitutes the stimulus to the visual system. However, consideration of a basic visual stimulus consisting of an isolated light source, which can vary in both intensity and wavelength, makes it clear that any visual stimulus will have a number of qualitatively different aspects. The appropriate mathematical structures for describing phenomena which vary both quantitatively and qualitatively are introduced in this chapter.

Definition of Vector Properties

In abstract terms, a VECTOR is a quantity which specifies both the length and the direction of a translation of a point through space. By convention, vectors are denoted by boldface type, e.g. **a, b, c**. A simple visual representation of a vector is provided by an arrow, with the tail representing the initial position of the point and the head representing the final position of the point, after the translation. The definition of vector addition and subtraction is in keeping with the concept of a vector as a translation, in that vector addition has been defined so that it corresponds to the effect of following one translation by another. The addition is carried out according to the parallelogram rule which is readily understood from Fig. 2.1. The rule states that if two vectors **a** and **b** form the adjacent sides of a parallelogram, then their sum is represented by the diagonal from the start of one vector to the finish of the other.

Subtraction of a vector **b** from a vector **a** is defined to be equivalent to adding to **a** a vector of the same length as **b**, but with the opposite direction. This definition ensures that subtracting a vector from itself gives a zero vector.

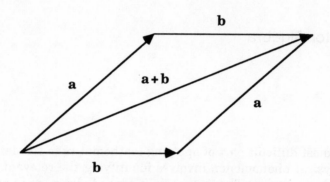

FIG. 2.1 The parallelogram rule for vector addition

The length of a vector, which is denoted by a pair of vertical lines on either side of the capital letter, e.g. |**a**|,|**b**|,|**c**|, can be altered independently of the direction of the vector by multiplication by a number. The number is referred to in this context as a SCALAR to signify that it has only magnitude whilst a vector has both magnitude and direction. Hence, if s is a scalar quantity then |s **a**| = s |**a**|. In order to distinguish them from vector quantities, scalar quantities will be written in italics. Besides vector addition, there are two further ways of combining vectors, which turn out to have many applications.

The SCALAR PRODUCT of two vectors **a** and **b** gives a scalar result which is proportional to the amount of the vector **b** that projects onto the direction of vector **a**. In Fig. 2.2 the amount of vector **b** that projects onto the direction of vector **a** is shown by the intersection of the dotted line with vector **a**. The actual value of the scalar product, which is denoted by **a·b**, is given by the definition:

a.b = |**a**||**b**|cos t

where t is the angle between **a** and **b**. Because the scalar product is proportional to the cosine of t, it becomes zero when the two vectors are perpendicular.

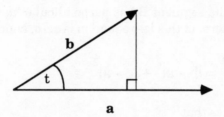

FIG. 2.2. The scalar product

The scalar product is useful for determining the angle between two vectors since:

$$\cos (\text{angle between } \mathbf{a} \text{ and } \mathbf{b}) = \frac{\mathbf{a}.\mathbf{b}}{|\mathbf{a}||\mathbf{b}|}$$

When the scalar product between two vectors is zero, then they are perpendicular to each other and are referred to as ORTHOGONAL VECTORS. It is also useful for determining the length of a vector since:

$$\mathbf{a}.\mathbf{a} = |\mathbf{a}||\mathbf{a}|$$

so

$$|\mathbf{a}| = \sqrt{\mathbf{a}.\mathbf{a}}$$

An example of the application of the scalar product is provided by the following proof of Pythagoras's theorem. Consider the diagram shown in Fig. 2.3. A, B and C are the three points at the corners of the triangle. Let $\mathbf{a}$, $\mathbf{b}$ and $\mathbf{c}$ be vectors to the three points and let $\mathbf{h}$ be a vector lying along the hypotenuse. It follows that:

$$\mathbf{h} = (\mathbf{b} - \mathbf{a}) - (\mathbf{c} - \mathbf{a})$$

so that

$$\mathbf{h}.\mathbf{h} = (\mathbf{b} - \mathbf{a}).(\mathbf{b} - \mathbf{a}) - 2(\mathbf{b} - \mathbf{a}).(\mathbf{c} - \mathbf{a}) + (\mathbf{c} - \mathbf{a}).(\mathbf{c} - \mathbf{a})$$

Since the line segment BA is perpendicular to the line segment AC the middle term of this last equation is zero, hence:

$$|\mathbf{h}|^2 = |\mathbf{b} - \mathbf{a}|^2 + |\mathbf{c} - \mathbf{a}|^2$$

which implies that

$$BC^2 = BA^2 + AC^2$$

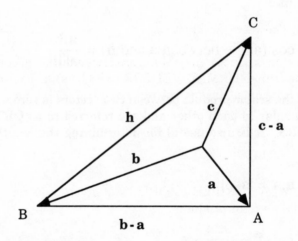

FIG. 2.3. Diagram of vectors used to prove Pythagoras's theorem

The VECTOR PRODUCT of two vectors **a** and **b** gives a vector which is perpendicular to both **a** and **b**, as shown in Fig. 2.4, and whose length is equal to the area of the parallelogram formed by **a** and **b**. Because it is inherently three - dimensional, the vector product is only defined for three - dimensional vectors. The result of forming the vector product of two vectors **a** and **b** is denoted by **a**∧**b** and is given by the definition:

$$\mathbf{a}{\wedge}\mathbf{b} = |\mathbf{a}||\mathbf{b}|\sin t \ \mathbf{n}$$

where **n** is a vector of unit length which is perpendicular to both **a** and **b** and t is the angle between **a** and **b**. The direction of the perpendicular vector is defined to be such that **a**∧**b** = - **b**∧**a**, so that for this operation, the order of the operands is important.

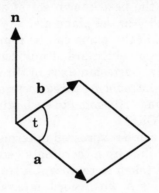

FIG. 2.4. The vector product

The vector product is useful for producing a unit vector **n**, referred to as the unit NORMAL VECTOR, which is perpendicular to the plane that includes the two vectors **a** and **b** since:

$$\mathbf{n} = \frac{\mathbf{a}^\wedge\mathbf{b}}{|\mathbf{a}^\wedge\mathbf{b}|}$$

The SCALAR TRIPLE PRODUCT is given by a combination of a scalar and a vector product:

$$[\mathbf{a}, \mathbf{b}, \mathbf{c}] = \mathbf{a}.(\mathbf{b}^\wedge\mathbf{c})$$

which results in a scalar quantity. The value of the scalar triple product is equal to the volume of the parallelpiped formed by the vectors **a**, **b** and **c**. The vector product **b**∧**c** gives the area spanned by the two vectors at the base of the parallelpiped, and the scalar product with the third vector **a** gives the product of this area with the perpendicular height of the parallelpiped. A necessary condition for three vectors to be coplanar is that their scalar triple product should be zero.

Vector Coordinates

The abstract concept of vectors highlights their important properties, but most applications require a definition of vectors in terms of fixed axes. Perhaps the best known set of axes are the Cartesian axes known as x and y in the plane and x, y and z in three dimensions. Cartesian axes in the plane can be represented by introducing two vectors e_1 and e_2, which are of unit length and orthogonal to each other. Similarly, Cartesian axes in three dimensional space can be represented by introducing three vectors e_1, e_2 and e_3, which are all of unit length and orthogonal to each other. These vectors are known as BASE VECTORS.

Any vector **a** can be expressed in terms of these base vectors in the way that is familiar from coordinate geometry, as shown in Fig. 2.5. The vector **a** is taken to represent a translation of a point from the origin to a point A with coordinates (a_1, a_2) in the plane and coordinates (a_1, a_2, a_3) in three dimensional space. In the plane, the procedure of placing the point at a distance a_1 along the x axis and at a distance a_2 along the y axis, corresponds to adding the vector $a_1\, e_1$ to the vector $a_2\, e_2$, so that one can write:

$$\mathbf{a} = a_1\, \mathbf{e}_1 + a_2\, \mathbf{e}_2$$

The corresponding expression for a vector in three dimensional axes is:

$$\mathbf{a} = a_1\, \mathbf{e}_1 + a_2\, \mathbf{e}_2 + a_3\, \mathbf{e}_3$$

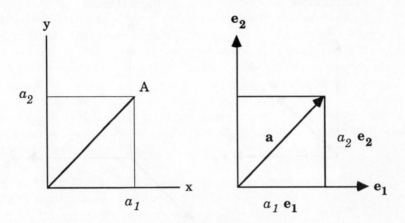

FIG. 2.5. Cartesian and vector coordinates

The procedure of adding together scalar multiples of a set of vectors is often encountered, and is referred to by the term LINEAR COMBINATION. The scalar multiples of the base vectors that are associated with a given vector are referred to as the COORDINATES of the vector, in keeping with the role of these numbers in coordinate geometry.

It is also convenient to specify vectors in terms of coordinates when the result of a scalar or vector product is required. For the scalar product, the cosines of the angles between e_1 and e_1, e_2 and e_2 and e_3 and e_3 are all equal to 1, whilst the cosines of the angles between e_1 and e_2, e_2 and e_3 and e_3 and e_1 are all equal to 0, so that in terms of coordinates the definition becomes:

$$\mathbf{a}.\mathbf{b} = a_1 b_1 + a_2 b_2 + a_3 b_3$$

Consideration of the vector product in terms of coordinates reveals that there are two possible directions for the e_3 vector as shown in Fig. 2.6. By convention the two different systems are referred to as a RIGHT HANDED and a LEFT HANDED system respectively.

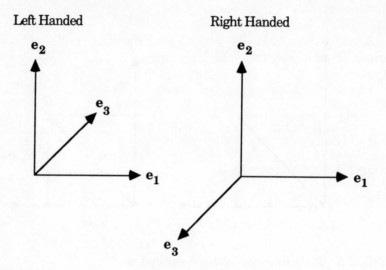

FIG. 2.6. Alternative systems of Cartesian base vectors

Once it is agreed that a given system is being used, one can then choose the direction of the vector **n** in the cross product to be such that the following rules are satisfied:

$$e_1{}^{\wedge}e_2 = - e_2{}^{\wedge}e_1 = e_3$$
$$e_2{}^{\wedge}e_3 = - e_3{}^{\wedge}e_2 = e_1$$
$$e_3{}^{\wedge}e_1 = - e_1{}^{\wedge}e_3 = e_2$$

and

$$e_1{}^{\wedge}e_1 = e_2{}^{\wedge}e_2 = e_3{}^{\wedge}e_3 = 0$$

so that in terms of coordinates:

$$\mathbf{a}^{\wedge}\mathbf{b} = (a_2b_3 - a_3b_2)\mathbf{e_1} - (a_1b_3 - a_3b_1)\mathbf{e_2} - (a_1b_2 - a_2b_1)\mathbf{e_3}$$

Summary

A vector is a quantity which specifies both the length and the direction of a translation through space, and is denoted by boldface type.

The two fundamental vector operations are the scalar product:

$$\mathbf{a.b} = a_1 b_1 + a_2 b_2 + a_3 b_3$$

and the vector product:

$$\mathbf{a^{\wedge}b} =$$
$$(a_2 b_3 - a_3 b_2)\mathbf{e_1} - (a_1 b_3 - a_3 b_1)\mathbf{e_2} - (a_1 b_2 - a_2 b_1)\mathbf{e_3}$$

CHAPTER 3

Matrix Algebra

Given that the approach of this book is to follow the changes in the
visual stimulus that occur along the visual pathway, the most
important mathematical tool is the one used to describe these
changes. This chapter introduces the mathematical structures
needed to describe changes between vectors.

Linear Transformations

The vector concept becomes more useful when it is tied in with a
description of the ways in which combinations of vectors can change
together. The simplest type of change is that associated with a
LINEAR TRANSFORMATION, which has two defining properties.
Let T be a linear transformation then:

$$T(\mathbf{u}_1 + \mathbf{u}_2) = T(\mathbf{u}_1) + T(\mathbf{u}_2)$$

for every pair of vectors $\mathbf{u}_1$ and $\mathbf{u}_2$, and

$$T(u\,\mathbf{u}) = u\,T(\mathbf{u})$$

for every scalar u and every vector $\mathbf{u}$.

The actual calculation of the transformation of each vector is carried out in terms of the coordinates of the vector. If a vector $\mathbf{u}$ in a vector space with base vectors $\mathbf{u_1}$, $\mathbf{u_2}$, ... $\mathbf{u_n}$ is transformed into a vector $\mathbf{v}$ in a vector space with base vectors $\mathbf{v_1}$, $\mathbf{v_2}$, ... $\mathbf{v_m}$, then:

$$\mathbf{u} = u_1\,\mathbf{u_1} + u_2\,\mathbf{u_2} + ... + u_n\,\mathbf{u_n}$$

and

$$T(\mathbf{u}) = \mathbf{v} = v_1\,\mathbf{v_1} + v_2\,\mathbf{v_2} + ... + v_m\,\mathbf{v_m}$$

But as the transformation is linear, it is also true that:

$$T(\mathbf{u}) = u_1\,T(\mathbf{u_1}) + u_2\,T(\mathbf{u_2}) + ... + u_n\,T(\mathbf{u_n})$$

and the transformations of each of the base vectors $\mathbf{u_1}$, $\mathbf{u_2}$, ... $\mathbf{u_n}$ can also be expressed in terms of $\mathbf{v_1}$, $\mathbf{v_2}$, ... $\mathbf{v_m}$. The key to keeping track of all the scalar constants involved is the introduction of a second subscript which specifies which base vector $\mathbf{u_i}$ is being referred to. The coordinates v_1, v_2, ... v_m which specify $T(\mathbf{u})$ in terms of the base vectors $\mathbf{v_1}$, $\mathbf{v_2}$, ... $\mathbf{v_m}$ are replaced by a set of scalars denoted by t_{1i}, t_{2i}, ... t_{mi}. The subscript i identifies the base vector $\mathbf{u_i}$ which is being expressed in terms of $\mathbf{v_1}$, $\mathbf{v_2}$, ... $\mathbf{v_m}$. Using this approach, the effect of the linear transformation T on a vector $\mathbf{u}$ can be defined by a set of linear equations:

$$u_1\,T(\mathbf{u_1}) = u_1\,(t_{11}\,\mathbf{v_1} + t_{21}\,\mathbf{v_2} + ... + t_{m1}\,\mathbf{v_m})$$

$$u_2\,T(\mathbf{u_2}) = u_2\,(t_{12}\,\mathbf{v_1} + t_{22}\,\mathbf{v_2} + ... + t_{m2}\,\mathbf{v_m})$$

$$...$$

$$u_n\,T(\mathbf{u_n}) = u_n\,(t_{1n}\,\mathbf{v_1} + t_{2n}\,\mathbf{v_2} + ... + t_{mn}\,\mathbf{v_m})$$

Equating the coefficients of $\mathbf{v_1}$, $\mathbf{v_2}$, ... $\mathbf{v_m}$ in this set of linear equations with the coordinates v_1, v_2, ... v_m which specify $T(\mathbf{u})$, gives a set of equations which specify the relation between the coordinates of the vectors $\mathbf{u}$ and $\mathbf{v}$:

$$v_1 = t_{11}u_1 + t_{12}u_2 + \dots + t_{1n}u_n$$

$$v_2 = t_{21}u_1 + t_{22}u_2 + \dots + t_{2n}u_n$$

$$\dots\dots\dots\dots\dots\dots\dots\dots\dots\dots\dots\dots$$

$$v_m = t_{m1}u_1 + t_{m2}u_2 + \dots + t_{mn}u_n$$

The set of scalar values $t_{11}, t_{12}, \dots t_{mn}$ can be written as an array with m rows and n columns, referred to as a MATRIX. Matrices are denoted by capital letters in italics, and the individual scalar values are referred to as elements of the matrix and are denoted by lower case letters in italics. The element in the ith row and j^{th} column of a matrix T is given the label t_{ij}. The contents of a matrix are enclosed in square brackets, so the set of scalars $t_{11}, t_{12}, \dots t_{mn}$ can be written as a matrix T where:

$$T = \begin{bmatrix} t_{11} & t_{12} & . & t_{1n} \\ t_{21} & t_{22} & . & t_{2n} \\ . & . & . & . \\ t_{m1} & t_{m2} & . & t_{mn} \end{bmatrix}$$

If the coordinates of the vectors **v** and **u** are written as matrices with one column then the linear equations which describe the relation between the coordinates $v_1, v_2, \dots v_m$ and $u_1, u_2, \dots u_n$ can be succinctly written as a single matrix equation:

$$v = Tu$$

If a linear transformation specified by a matrix B is applied after a linear transformation specified by a matrix A then the combination of linear transformations is itself a linear transformation, the effect of which can be described by a single matrix BA. The matrix BA is referred to as the MATRIX PRODUCT of B and A. The elements of the matrix BA can be evaluated by treating each column of the product matrix as an instance of a matrix equation. Thus, the element in the ith row and j^{th} column of BA is given by the scalar product of the vector corresponding to the ith row of B with the vector corresponding to the jth column of A. In practice, this sort of routine computation can be dealt with by invoking a mathematics package.

Change of Basis

A particular type of linear transformation arises when one set of n base vectors is changed into another set of n base vectors. In this case individual vectors are not changed, only their coordinates. Because the number of base vectors is the same before and after the linear transformation each vector $\mathbf{u_1}$', $\mathbf{u_2}$', ... $\mathbf{u_n}$' of the new set of base vectors can be described as a linear combination of the original vectors $\mathbf{u_1}$, $\mathbf{u_2}$, ... $\mathbf{u_n}$ and these linear combinations can be written as a matrix equation:

$$\begin{bmatrix} \mathbf{u_1}' \\ \mathbf{u_2}' \\ . \\ \mathbf{u_n}' \end{bmatrix} = A \begin{bmatrix} \mathbf{u_1} \\ \mathbf{u_2} \\ . \\ \mathbf{u_n} \end{bmatrix}$$

When n = 2 the base vectors span the plane and the matrix equation becomes:

$$\begin{bmatrix} \mathbf{u_1}' \\ \mathbf{u_2}' \end{bmatrix} = \begin{bmatrix} a_{11} & a_{12} \\ a_{21} & a_{22} \end{bmatrix} \begin{bmatrix} \mathbf{u_1} \\ \mathbf{u_2} \end{bmatrix}$$

If the coordinates of a vector $\mathbf{u}$ are u_1, u_2 in the $\mathbf{u_1}$, $\mathbf{u_2}$ system of base vectors and u_1', u_2' in the $\mathbf{u_1}$', $\mathbf{u_2}$' system of base vectors, then as both sets of coordinates refer to the same vector it holds that:

$$u_1 \mathbf{u_1} = u_1' \mathbf{u_1}' = u_1' a_{11} \mathbf{u_1} + u_1' a_{12} \mathbf{u_2}$$

$$u_2 \mathbf{u_2} = u_2' \mathbf{u_2}' = u_2' a_{21} \mathbf{u_1} + u_2' a_{22} \mathbf{u_2}$$

Hence the relationship between the coordinates of the vector in the two systems of base vectors is given by:

$$u_1 = a_{11}u_1' + a_{21}u_2'$$

$$u_2 = a_{12}u_1' + a_{22}u_2'$$

so that the coordinates are related by a matrix which is obtained by swopping the rows and columns of the matrix A describing the base vectors $\mathbf{u_1}'$ and $\mathbf{u_2}'$ as linear combinations of the $\mathbf{u_1}$ and $\mathbf{u_2}$ base vectors.

A similar result holds for transformations between three dimensional sets of base vectors. In this case the matrix equation which specifies $\mathbf{u_1}'$, $\mathbf{u_2}'$ and $\mathbf{u_3}'$ as linear combinations of $\mathbf{u_1}$, $\mathbf{u_2}$ and $\mathbf{u_3}$ is:

$$\begin{bmatrix} \mathbf{u_1}' \\ \mathbf{u_2}' \\ \mathbf{u_3}' \end{bmatrix} = \begin{bmatrix} a_{11} & a_{12} & a_{13} \\ a_{21} & a_{22} & a_{23} \\ a_{31} & a_{32} & a_{33} \end{bmatrix} \begin{bmatrix} \mathbf{u_1} \\ \mathbf{u_2} \\ \mathbf{u_3} \end{bmatrix}$$

and the coordinates are such that:

$$u_1\,\mathbf{u_1} = u_1'\,\mathbf{u_1}' = u_1'a_{11}\,\mathbf{u_1} + u_1'a_{12}\,\mathbf{u_2} + u_1'a_{13}\,\mathbf{u_3}$$

$$u_2\,\mathbf{u_2} = u_2'\,\mathbf{u_2}' = u_2'a_{21}\,\mathbf{u_1} + u_2'a_{22}\,\mathbf{u_2} + u_3'a_{23}\,\mathbf{u_3}$$

$$u_3\,\mathbf{u_3} = u_3'\,\mathbf{u_3}' = u_3'a_{31}\,\mathbf{u_1} + u_3'a_{32}\,\mathbf{u_2} + u_3'a_{33}\,\mathbf{u_3}$$

equating the coordinates of each of the base vectors $\mathbf{u_1}$, $\mathbf{u_2}$ and $\mathbf{u_3}$ gives the relationship between the coordinates:

$$u_1 = a_{11}u_1' + a_{21}u_1' + a_{31}u_1'$$

$$u_2 = a_{12}u_2' + a_{22}u_2' + a_{32}u_2'$$

$$u_3 = a_{13}u_3' + a_{23}u_3' + a_{33}u_3'$$

The matrix obtained from a matrix A by writing the rows as columns and vice versa is referred to as the TRANSPOSE of A and is denoted by A^T. In terms of individual elements $a_{ij}{}^T = a_{ji}$. With this notation, the equation for the transformation of coordinates can be written as:

$$u = A^T u'$$

As the matrix A corresponds to a change of basis the transformation can be reversed and so:

$$u' = A^{T\text{-}1} u$$

where the INVERSE MATRIX $A^{T\text{-}1}$ is such that:

$$A^{T\text{-}1} A^T = \begin{bmatrix} 1 & 0 & 0 & \dots & 0 \\ 0 & 1 & 0 & \dots & 0 \\ . & . & . & \dots & . \\ 0 & 0 & 0 & \dots & 1 \end{bmatrix}$$

If B is a matrix which describes the transformation of coordinates under a change of basis and T is the matrix of a linear transformation for which m = n then

$$u = Bu' \quad \text{and} \quad v' = B^{-1}v$$

so $v = Tu$ implies that:

$$Bv' = TBu'$$

which gives a new matrix equation:

$$v' = B^{-1}TBu' = Su'$$

The matrices S and $B^{-1}TB$ both describe the same linear transformation, only with respect to different bases, and are referred to as SIMILAR matrices. The significance of similar matrices is that by a suitable choice of basis the linear transformation T can be given its simplest form S, which has a diagonal matrix representation.

The appropriate basis can be found by considering vectors which do not change direction under the transformation, and so satisfy the equation:

$$Tu = \lambda u$$

A vector which satisfies this equation is referred to as an EIGENVECTOR of the linear transformation and the scalar constant λ is referred to as the EIGENVALUE of the vector.

If T is represented by an n by n matrix and one can find n different eigenvectors then one can form the required n by n change of basis matrix B by writing the eigenvectors into the columns of the matrix. It follows from the definition of an eigenvector that:

$$TB = BS$$

where the elements of S are all zero except for the elements along the diagonal s_{11} to s_{nn} which are equal to the eigenvalues associated with the successive columns of B. Hence, with the change of basis defined by the matrix B the linear transformation defined by T takes on the simple form $S = B^{-1}TB$ where:

$$S = \begin{bmatrix} \lambda_1 & 0 & \cdots & 0 \\ 0 & \lambda_2 & \cdots & 0 \\ 0 & 0 & \cdots & 0 \\ 0 & 0 & \cdots & \lambda_n \end{bmatrix}$$

Summary

An m by n matrix A is an array of numbers with m rows and n columns which defines a linear transformation from one set of base vectors to another.

The matrix product BA describes the effect of applying the linear transformation defined by the matrix A followed by the linear transformation defined by the matrix B.

The matrix of a linear transformation can be simplified by an appropriate choice of the base vectors used to describe the transformation. An eigenvector of a matrix A does not change its direction when multiplied by A, only its length. If n eigenvectors can be found for an n by n matrix A, then a matrix B which specifies the required change of basis can be formed by writing the eigenvectors into the columns of B. The similar matrices $S = B^{-1}AB$ and A both represent the same linear transformation but S has a diagonal form.

CHAPTER 4

Gaussian Optics

The first stage of visual processing involves the formation of the retinal images. In this chapter, it is shown how 2x2 matrices can be used to calculate the properties of the image formed by an optical system.

Geometrical Optics

The Gaussian approach to optics is based on the simplifying assumption that all the rays of light arising from a given point intersect at another point after passing through an optical system. The set of points before the refractions is referred to as the OBJECT SPACE and the set of points formed by the refractions is referred to as the IMAGE SPACE. A point in object space and its associated image point are referred to as CONJUGATE POINTS.

The simplest form of refracting surfaces are ones whose surfaces form a portion of a sphere. Such refracting surfaces are usually arranged so that their centres of curvature lie along a straight line. This straight line is referred to as the OPTICAL AXIS of the optical system. The locations of the surfaces are specified with respect to the point where the surface intersects with the optical axis, which is referred to as the VERTEX of the surface.

The method for understanding a complex system of refracting surfaces, which was introduced by Gauss, involves replacing the system with a simpler, but equivalent system. Rays entering an optical system parallel to the optical axis will converge to a focal point in image space, as shown in Fig. 4.1. The convergence of the rays is equivalent to that of a single lens located at the plane P' where the fan of rays converging onto the focal point intersects with the parallel rays entering the optical system. This plane is referred to as the PRINCIPAL PLANE in image space. The lens located at the principal plane must have a focal length equal to the distance f' between the principal plane and the focal point of the whole system, and for the purposes of this analysis is considered to be a 'thin' lens, that is, one with negligible width.

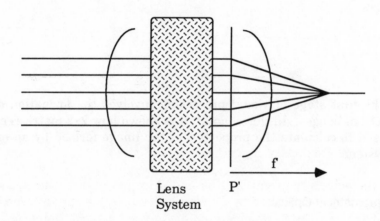

Lens   P'
System

FIG. 4.1. Location of the principal plane in image space

Clearly, there is a corresponding principal plane P in object space with focal length f such that rays coming from the focal point of the system in object space will emerge parallel after refraction by the equivalent thin lens. These two principal planes are conjugate to each other, for if one specifies a point X on the principal plane P by the intersection of a ray parallel to the optical axis with a ray from the focal point in object space, as shown in Fig. 4.2, then after passing through the optical system the two rays intersect at the point X' on the principal plane P'. According to the Gaussian approach, all rays through a point X in object space must pass through its image X' in image space, so the point of intersection of a ray with the image plane will be independent of the initial direction of the ray. Hence the height h' of the image point above the optical axis depends only on the height h of the object point above the optical axis and one can define the LINEAR MAGNIFICATION m to be equal to the ratio h'/h. Since h = h' in Fig. 4.2, it follows that a further distinguishing feature of the principal planes is that they have unit linear magnification between them.

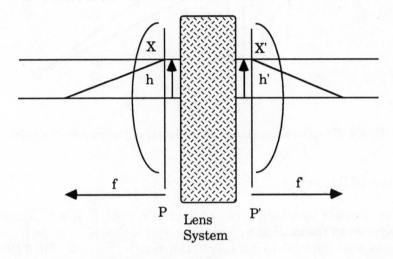

FIG. 4.2. Conjugacy of principal planes

As well as the focal lengths and principal planes, the equivalent optical system devised by Gauss also requires the specification of the NODAL POINTS, which are defined to be a pair of conjugate points on the optical axis. Their characteristic property is that a ray intersecting with one nodal point makes the same angle with the optical axis when it passes through the other nodal point. The image of any point can then be constructed graphically by tracing two rays, one parallel to the optical axis, and one through the nodal points, as shown in Fig. 4.3. The next two sections will tackle the problem of how to calculate the locations of the Gaussian constants of an optical system from its component parts.

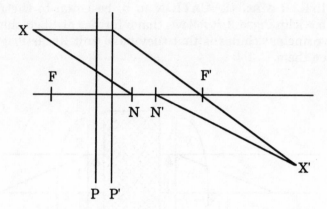

FIG. 4.3. Graphical construction for locating the image of a point.

Paraxial Raytracing

The amount by which a ray of light is refracted at a lens surface depends on the amount by which the light is slowed down as it passes from one material to another. The relative velocity for different materials can be characterised by the refractive index p which is unity for air and 1.33 for water. Let the angle of incidence i be the angle between the incident ray and the normal to the refracting surface and the angle of refraction i' be the angle between the refracted ray and the normal. Then the laws governing the refracted ray are as follows:

1) The incident ray, refracted ray and normal all lie in the same plane

2) sin i/sin i'=(n medium of refracted ray/n medium of incident ray)

The second constraint is known as Snell's law and describes how, when a light ray passes from a rare into a dense medium, it is bent or 'refracted', towards the normal to the interface, and how it is bent away when passing from a dense to a rare medium.

In geometrical analyses of raytracing it is customary to assume that the ray passes from left to right in the diagram. In keeping with this assumption, distances are measured as positive from left to right.

Hence a convex lens will be specified by a positive radius and a concave lens by a negative radius. A further convention is that the angle that a ray makes with the optical axis is specified as positive in an anti - clockwise direction. Hence in Fig. 4.4a, a ray makes a positive angle with the optical axis and is directed towards a convex lens. In Fig. 4.4b, the angle is negative and the lens is concave.

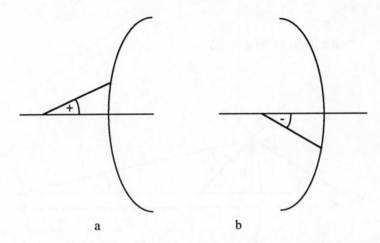

a   b

FIG. 4.4. Sign conventions for raytracing a) Ray at an anti - clockwise (positive) angle intersecting with a convex (positive radius) surface. b) Ray at a clockwise (negative) angle intersecting with a concave (negative radius) surface.

The analytical treatment of an axial optical system is considerably simplified by considering only PARAXIAL RAYS, which lie close to the axis of the optical system. In the paraxial case, trigonometric relations become simplified, as for any angle a :

$$\sin a = a$$
$$\cos a = 1$$
$$\tan a = a$$

Applying the paraxial relations to Snell's law, one obtains the equation:

$$ni = n'i'$$

This equation can be rewritten in terms of the angles a and a', which are the angles that the incident and refracted rays make with the optical axis, and the angle b that the normal associated with the ray makes with the optical axis, as shown in Fig. 4.5. The substitution is not difficult, since it only involves expressing i as the third angle of a triangle, but it does require that the sign convention for the angles is adhered to. After the substitution the equation describing Snell's law becomes:

$$n(a + b) = n'(a' + b)$$

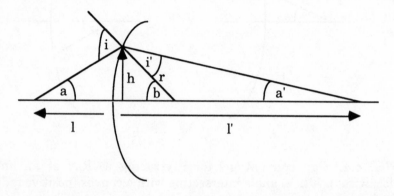

FIG. 4.5. Variables involved in calculating the direction of a refracted ray

By application of the small angle approximation the angle b can in turn be expressed in terms of the height h of the ray above the optical axis and the radius r of the lens surface. The equation for Snell's law then becomes:

$$n(a + \frac{h}{r}) = n'(a' + \frac{h}{r})$$

which is equivalent to the equation

$$n'a' = na - \frac{(n' - n)h}{r} = na - dh$$

where d = (n' - n)/r, which is a quantity referred to as the POWER of the lens.

The significance of the power of a lens is revealed by a further application of the paraxial assumption so that the previous equation becomes:

$$\frac{nh}{l} = \frac{n'h}{l'} - dh$$

where l is the distance from the lens to the point where the incident ray leaves the optical axis and l' is the distance from the lens to the point where the refracted ray hits the optical axis. Both these distances are measured with respect to the lens vertex. Finally, cancelling out h gives the basic equation of refraction:

$$\frac{n}{l} = \frac{n'}{l'} - d$$

If the incident ray is parallel to the optical axis then the term n/l is effectively zero and the distance l' = n'/d. If the medium of the refracted ray is air then n' = 1 so that the power is the reciprocal of the focal length of the lens in air. In order to be able to compare the powers of different optical systems, power is specified by the reciprocal of the focal length in air given in metres. The unit of power is the DIOPTRE, so that a system with a focal length in air of one metre has a power of one dioptre. To be consistent with this definition, the radius of curvature of a lens surface must be specified in metres, when calculating the power of the lens according to the formula d = (n' - n)/r.

The description of the path between two refracting surfaces depends on the fact that the angle that the ray makes with the optical axis is unchanged, as shown in Fig. 4.6. If the distance between the surfaces is t then:

$$h' = h + t(\tan a) = h + ta$$

since the ray is paraxial.

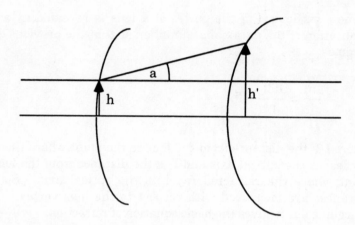

FIG. 4.6. Variables involved in calculating the translation of a ray between two surfaces.

Matrix Raytracing

The path of a ray through a sequence of refracting surfaces can be succinctly described in matrix notation. The algebra is simplified by expressing the distance along a ray divided by the refractive index of the ray as a single variable, referred to as the REDUCED DISTANCE. Such reduced distances will be denoted by capital letters so that t/n is equal to the reduced distance T.

Each ray is represented by a single column matrix:

$$\begin{bmatrix} na \\ h \end{bmatrix}$$

where h equals the height of the ray above the optical axis, a equals the angle that the ray makes with the optical axis and n is the refractive index of the medium that the ray is passing through.

The refraction of a ray at a surface can then be described by the matrix equation:

$$\begin{bmatrix} n'a' \\ h' \end{bmatrix} = \begin{bmatrix} 1 & -d \\ 0 & 1 \end{bmatrix} \begin{bmatrix} na \\ h \end{bmatrix}$$

and the translation of a ray between two surfaces can be described by the matrix equation:

$$\begin{bmatrix} n'a' \\ h' \end{bmatrix} = \begin{bmatrix} 1 & 0 \\ T & 1 \end{bmatrix} \begin{bmatrix} na \\ h \end{bmatrix}$$

where T is the reduced distance between the refracting surfaces.

The properties of a system of refracting surfaces can be encapsulated by the SYSTEM MATRIX of the system. The system matrix will be denoted by the capital letter S, and is given by the product of the sequence of refraction and translation matrices associated with the lens system. For a single lens, consisting of a pair of refracting surfaces, the sequence would be refraction - translation - refraction.

$$\begin{aligned} S &= \begin{bmatrix} 1 & -d_2 \\ 0 & 1 \end{bmatrix} \begin{bmatrix} 1 & 0 \\ T & 1 \end{bmatrix} \begin{bmatrix} 1 & -d_1 \\ 0 & 1 \end{bmatrix} \\[2mm] &= \begin{bmatrix} 1 & -d_2 \\ 0 & 1 \end{bmatrix} \begin{bmatrix} 1 & -d_1 \\ T & 1 - d_1 T \end{bmatrix} \\[2mm] &= \begin{bmatrix} 1 - d_2 T & -d_1 - d_2 + d_1 d_2 T \\ T & 1 - d_1 T \end{bmatrix} \end{aligned}$$

where d_1 is the power of the front surface of the lens, d_2 is the power of the back surface of the lens, t is the distance between the two refracting surfaces and n' is the refractive index of the lens and T = t/n'

The system matrix is used in calculations which involve determining the relation between a pair of conjugate points. The transformation of an object point into an image point Q can be described by the matrix sequence translation - lens system - translation, corresponding to the path shown in Fig. 4.7.

$$Q = T'ST = \begin{bmatrix} 1 & 0 \\ L' & 1 \end{bmatrix} \begin{bmatrix} s_{11} & s_{12} \\ s_{21} & s_{22} \end{bmatrix} \begin{bmatrix} 1 & 0 \\ -L & 1 \end{bmatrix}$$

$$= \begin{bmatrix} 1 & 0 \\ L' & 1 \end{bmatrix} \begin{bmatrix} s_{11} - s_{12} L & s_{12} \\ s_{21} - s_{22} L & s_{22} \end{bmatrix}$$

$$= \begin{bmatrix} s_{11} - s_{12} L & s_{12} \\ (s_{11} - s_{12} L)L' + (s_{21} - s_{22} L) & s_{12} L' + s_{22} \end{bmatrix}$$

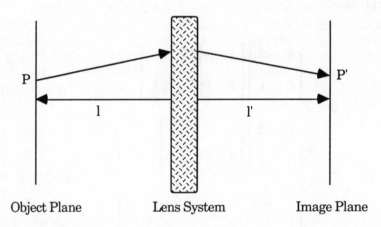

Object Plane   Lens System   Image Plane

FIG. 4.7. Object - Image transformation

The constraint that the linear magnification m between two conjugate points should be independent of the direction of the incoming ray implies that h'/h does not depend on the angle of the ray a so the element $q_{21} = 0$. It follows immediately that m = q_{22} = h'/h.

The matrix can be simplified still more by an application of some further matrix algebra. The DETERMINANT of a matrix is a function of the elements of a matrix which becomes zero if the row vectors which make up the matrix are linearly dependent. In the case of a 2 x 2 matrix, the value of the determinant is equal to the area of the parallelogram spanned by the row vectors. Let A be a 2 x 2 matrix, then the determinant of A , which is denoted by $|A|$ is given by:

$$|A| = a_{11}a_{22} - a_{21}a_{12}$$

The property of determinants that is useful in this context is that the determinant of the product of two matrices is equal to the product of the determinants of the individual matrices. Let A and B be n x n matrices then:

$$|AB| = |A| \, |B|$$

In the simple case of 2 x 2 matrices, this equality can be proved by expanding out both sides into the elements of the matrices according to the definition of the determinant and then equating terms.

Since the determinants of both the refraction and translation matrices are unity, and since the matrix Q, which describes the transformation between object and image planes, is formed by the product of only refraction and translation matrices, it must be that $|Q| = 1$. This can only be so if $1/m = q_{11}$. Hence, the matrix Q can be simplified to:

$$Q = \begin{bmatrix} 1/m & s_{12} \\ 0 & m \end{bmatrix}$$

where m is the linear magnification between the two planes and s_{12} is the power of the optical system.

The constraint that $q_{21} = 0$ gives the equation:

$$- s_{12} \, LL' + s_{11} \, L' - s_{22} \, L + s_{21} = 0$$

and this equation can be rearranged to give the relations between the distances to the conjugate planes:

$$L' = - \frac{s_{21} - s_{22} \, L}{s_{11} - s_{12} \, L} = - \frac{s_{21} - s_{22} \, L}{q_{11}} = - (s_{21} - s_{22} \, L) \, m$$

and

$$L = \frac{s_{21} + s_{11} \, L'}{s_{22} + s_{12} \, L'} = \frac{s_{21} + s_{11} \, L'}{q_{22}} = \frac{s_{21} + s_{11} \, L'}{m}$$

Schematic eyes

The main refracting surfaces in the eye are located at the cornea, which is the transparent membrane that forms the bulge at the front of the eye, and at the crystalline lens. The refractive indices of excised corneas and lenses, and of aqueous and vitreous humours have been measured directly. The index of the lens changes smoothly throughout its width and so cannot be accurately represented by a single value. However, for simplicity, this index is set to a value that ensures that the overall schematic eye is in focus for rays entering it in parallel.

The most direct way to determine the curvature of the cornea is to use a micromanipulator to probe the surface, and then to fit a sphere to the data. The curvature of the back of the cornea has usually been estimated by assuming that it is concentric with the anterior cornea. The difference between the two radii is obtained by measuring the thickness of the cornea. The radius of curvature of the back and front of the lens can also be determined by using a probe to map the surfaces of the dissected out lens.

The radius of curvature of the retina can be obtained by measuring the radius of the back of an excised eye. On the assumption that the outside of the eye and the retina are concentric, the distance between the retina and the outside of the eye can be estimated from photographs of cross - sections of the eye, after taking into account the shrinkage of the sectioned tissue.

As the distance between the cornea and the back of the eye can be determined from external measurements of the eye, it only remains to specify the position of the lens. Typically this is done from photographs of sections of the eye.

More accurate estimates of the parameters of a schematic eye can be made by extensive use of non - invasive optometric investigations.

Details of such techniques can be found in Le Grand (1945), and the values given in Tables 4.1 - 4.3 are taken from this source.

TABLE 4.1 Radii of curvature of the optical surfaces of a human schematic eye (in millimetres)

Anterior Cornea	Posterior Cornea	Anterior Lens	Posterior Lens	Retina
7.8	6.5	10.2	-6.0	-12.0

TABLE 4.2 Positions of the optical surfaces of a human schematic eye (in millimetres)

Anterior Cornea	Posterior Cornea	Anterior Lens	Posterior Lens	Retina
0.0	0.55	3.6	7.6	24.2

TABLE 4.3 Refractive indices of the optical media of a human schematic eye

Cornea	Aqueous	Equivalent Lens	Vitreous
1.376	1.336	1.42	1.336

Given the parameters of the surfaces of the schematic eye it is straightforward to calculate the Gaussian constants. The system matrix is obtained by multiplying together matrices representing the refracting surfaces and the translations between them.

$$S = \begin{bmatrix} 0.904 & -59.8858 \\ 0.0054 & 0.7452 \end{bmatrix}$$

Example Calculation: The system matrix of a schematic eye for the cat

The radii of curvature, positions and refractive indices of the components of a schematic eye for the cat were determined by Vakkur, Bishop and Kozak (1963) and Vakkur and Bishop (1963), and their values are given in Tables 4.4 - 4.6.

TABLE 4.4 Radii of curvature of the optical surfaces of a cat schematic eye (in millimetres)

Anterior Cornea	Posterior Cornea	Anterior Lens	Posterior Lens	Retina
8.57	7.89	7.2	-8.05	-12.03

TABLE 4.5 Positions of the optical surfaces of a cat schematic eye (in millimetres)

Anterior Cornea	Posterior Cornea	Anterior Lens	Posterior Lens	Retina
0.0	0.68	5.2	13.7	21.83

TABLE 4.6 Refractive indices of the optical media of cat schematic eye

Cornea	Aqueous	Equivalent Lens	Vitreous
1.376	1.336	1.5544	1.336

The calculation of the system matrix for the schematic eye can be done using the speadsheet Wingz. Listed below are the matrices which describe each component of the schematic eye, and these have to be typed into the spreadsheet. The way in which the system matrix is built up is shown alongside the component matrices. The first matrix product is formed by multiplying the anterior cornea refraction matrix by the corneal translation matrix. The next product matrix is formed by multiplying the first product matrix by the posterior cornea refraction matrix, and so on. The product matrices are formed simply by selecting the multiplier first, the multiplicand second, the destination of the product third, and then choosing the matrix multiply option from the menu.

COMPONENT MATRICES   PRODUCT MATRICES

Refraction at Anterior Corneal Surface

1	-43.87398
0	1

Translation through Cornea

1	0		1.00000	-43.87398
0.00049	1		0.00049	0.97850

Refraction at Posterior Corneal Surface

1	5.06971		1.00248	-38.91326
0	1		0.00049	0.97850

Translation through Aqueous

1.00000	0.00000		1.00248	-38.91326
0.00338	1.00000		0.00388	0.84697

Refraction at Anterior Lens Surface

1	-30.33333		0.88484	-64.60483
0	1		0.00388	0.84697

Translation through Lens

1	0		0.88484	-64.60483
0.00547	1		0.00872	0.49359

Refraction at Posterior Lens Surface

1	-27.13043		0.64830	-77.99604
0	1		0.00872	0.49359

This final matrix product of all the component matrices is the system matrix for cat schematic eye.

Since the focal point in object space is on the optical axis and all rays leaving from it emerge from the eye in parallel, h = 0 and a'n' = 0 so $q_{11} = s_{11} - s_{12}$ F = 0. It follows that:

$$F = \frac{s_{11}}{s_{12}} = -0.0151$$

and by a similar argument

$$F' = - \frac{s_{22}}{s_{12}} = 0.0124$$

To convert these values into distances in metres, they must be multiplied by the refractive index of the medium of the space in which they lie. In the case of F the medium is air and in the case of F' the medium is the vitreous. One also has to remember that the distance to F' is reckoned from the vertex of the last surface of the optical system, which in this case is the back of the lens.

For the principal planes $m = 1 = q_{22} = 1/q_{11}$ so

$$P = \frac{1 - s_{11}}{s_{12}} = 0.0015$$

$$P' = \frac{s_{22} - 1}{s_{12}} = -0.0043$$

Finally, for the nodal points $h = h' = 0$ and $an = a'n'$ so $q_{11} = n'/n$. When the object space and image space have the same refractive indices then the positions of the nodal points are equal to the positions of the principal planes. For the schematic eye, the refractive indices are unequal so:

$$N = \frac{\frac{n'}{n} - s_{11}}{s_{12}} = 0.0072$$

$$N' = \frac{s_{22} - \dfrac{n'}{n}}{s_{12}} = -0.0001$$

A scale diagram of the schematic eye is shown in Fig. 4.8.

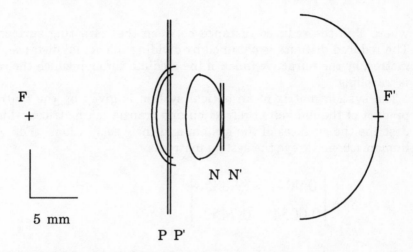

FIG. 4.8. Cross - section of the schematic eye, with the positions of the principal planes and the nodal points marked by long and short vertical lines respectively.

Summary

Paraxial rays are those which lie close to the optical axis of the system. Each ray can be described by a vector [na, h] where n is the refractive index of the medium through which the ray is passing, a is the angle which the ray makes with the optical axis and h is the height of the ray above the axis.

The refraction of a ray at a spherical surface is described by the refraction matrix:

$$\begin{bmatrix} 1 & -d \\ 0 & 1 \end{bmatrix}$$

where d is the power of the surface in dioptres.

The translation of a ray between two refracting surfaces is described by the translation matrix:

$$\begin{bmatrix} 1 & 0 \\ T & 1 \end{bmatrix}$$

where T is the reduced distance between the refracting surfaces. The reduced distance is obtained by dividing the actual distance, in metres, by the refractive index of the medium through which the ray is travelling.

The system matrix of an optical system is given by the matrix product of the individual refraction and translation matrices which describe the surfaces of the system and their separations. For the human schematic eye the system matrix is:

$$S = \begin{bmatrix} 0.904 & -59.8858 \\ 0.0054 & 0.7452 \end{bmatrix}$$

The reduced distance L of an object point from the front vertex of the optical system is related to the reduced distance L' of its image from the back vertex of the optical system by the conjugacy relations:

$$L' = -\frac{s_{21} - s_{22} L}{s_{11} - s_{12} L}$$

and

$$L = \frac{s_{21} + s_{11} L'}{s_{22} + s_{12} L'}$$

CHAPTER 5

Visual Optics

Gaussian optics is ideally suited to handling images which are in focus, but objects in a three - dimensional world are frequently out of focus. In this chapter the theory of Gaussian optics is used to determine the blur and visual directions of out of focus images.

Blur

The geometrical approach to optics can be extended to describe the blur of the retinal image, by considering the blurred image of a point. Rays from the point will hit the edge of the pupil and converge to a point focus and if the retina is not located at the focus then the cross section of the bundle of rays will be circular. This circular image of a point is referred to as the BLUR CIRCLE.

The size of the image of a point on the retina depends on the size of the pupil, which is located at the lens vertex. The image of the pupil which is conjugate to the actual pupil with respect to the cornea is referred to as the ENTRANCE PUPIL. This is the image of the pupil that one sees when one looks into an eye. The image of the pupil which is conjugate to the actual pupil with respect to the lens is referred to as the EXIT PUPIL. The entrance and exit pupils are conjugate to each other with respect to the whole eye.

The diameter of the blur circle on the retina associated with an object point P can be calculated from the paths of the rays which hit the extremities of the pupil; these rays are shown in Fig. 5.1. In the figure the diameter of the exit pupil is given by the length of the line CD. By similar triangles:

$$\frac{CD}{AB} = \frac{CP'}{AP'} = \frac{x'}{f' + x'}$$

so

$$CD = AB \cdot \frac{x'}{f' + x'}$$

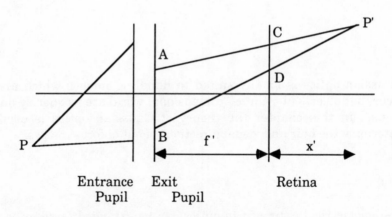

FIG. 5.1. Calculation of the size of the blur circle

The system matrices for the cornea and the lens can be used to calculate the locations of the entrance and exit pupils of the eye respectively, by application of the conjugacy relations. In the case of the entrance pupil, the system matrix for the cornea is:

$$S = \begin{bmatrix} 1.0025 & -42.17 \\ 0.0004 & 0.9807 \end{bmatrix}$$

As the iris lies along the surface of the lens, the position of the pupil is approximately equal to that of the anterior lens vertex, and the conjugate object plane is located 0.00249 metres behind the back vertex of the cornea.

The system matrix for the lens is:

$$S = \begin{bmatrix} 0.9606 & -21.9105 \\ 0.0028 & 0.9768 \end{bmatrix}$$

The distance of the iris from the anterior vertex of the lens is zero, so the conjugate image plane is located -0.0039 metres from the vertex at the back of the lens. With respect to the anterior vertex of the eye, the entrance pupil lies 3.04 millimetres behind it and the exit pupil lies 3.68 millimetres behind it, as shown in Fig. 5.2.

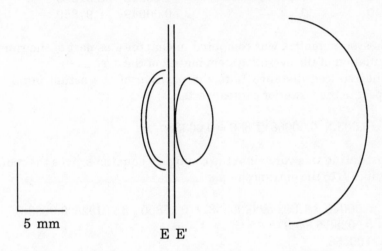

5 mm

E E'

FIG. 5.2 Human schematic eye with the locations of the entrance (E) and exit (E') pupils marked by vertical lines.

Example Calculation: Entrance and exit pupils of the cat eye

The system matrix of the cornea of the schematic eye of the cat can be calculated using Wingz, as in the example in chapter 4:

COMPONENT MATRICES   PRODUCT MATRICES

Refraction at Anterior Corneal Surface

1   -43.87398
0   1

Translation through Cornea

1   0   1.00000 -43.87398
0.00049   1   0.00049   0.97850

Refraction at Posterior Corneal Surface

1   5.06971   1.00248 -38.91326
0   1   0.00049   0.97850

This system matrix was computed in chapter 4 as part of the running calculation of the overall system matrix of the eye.

The reduced distance L' to the position of the actual pupil with respect to the posterior corneal vertex is:

L' = (0.0052 - 0.00068)/1.336 = 0.00338

Substituting this value into the conjugacy equations gives the reduced distance L to the entrance pupil:

L = (0.00049 + 1.00248*0.00338) / (0.97850 - 38.91326*0.00338)
  = 0.00388/0 84697
  = 0.00458

Since the refractive index of air is unity, L is equal to the distance behind the anterior corneal vertex of the entrance pupil. A corresponding calculation can be carried out to locate the exit pupil with respect to the lens.

COMPONENT MATRICES   PRODUCT MATRICES

Refraction at Anterior Lens Surface

1   -30.33333
0   1

Translation through Lens

1	0
0.005471	0.00547

1	-30.33333
0.83408	

Refraction at Posterior Lens Surface

1	-27.13043
0	1

0.85160	-52.96219
0.00547	0.83408

The position of the actual pupil is identical with the anterior lens vertex so:

$L = 0$

From the conjugacy relations it follows that:

$L' = -0.00547 / 0.8516 = -0.00642$

Therefore, the actual distance l to the exit pupil is

$l = -0.00642 * 1.336 = 0.00858$

From the anterior corneal vertex:

$l = 0.0137 - 0.00876 = 0.00512$

The linear magnification m between the entrance and exit pupils can be obtained directly from the matrix of the object plane to image plane transformation. $m = 77.99604 * 0.00642 + 0.49359 = 0.99$.

Helmholtz (1910) introduced a simple description of the blur of a step edge of unit luminance which follows from the observation that the intensity at a point q on the retina depends on the amount of the edge which is imaged within the blur circle centred at q, since every image point within this circle will itself have a blur circle that includes q. The area of the circle covered by the edge is given by the area of the segment of the circle which just touches the edge, plus an additional triangular portion. In Fig. 5.3, the hatched region represents the dark side of the edge and the stippled region corresponds to the additional triangular portion.

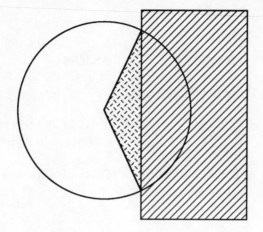

FIG. 5.3. Regions involved in calculation of the retinal light distribution of a step edge

If r denotes the radius of the blur circle then the area of the blur circle is πr^2 and the area of the segment containing the edge is wr^2 where w is half the angle subtended by the edge, as shown in Fig. 5.4. Since r cos w = - x, where x is the distance from the edge to the centre of the blur circle, it follows that w = arccos (- x / r). The area of the triangular portion of the segment is equal to $xy = x\sqrt{(r^2 - x^2)}$, where y is half the length of the edge which is contained in the circle. Hence the luminance distribution on the retina l(x) is given by the formula:

$$l(x) = r^2 \arccos - \frac{x}{r} + x \sqrt{r^2 - x^2}$$

and this function is plotted in Fig. 5.5

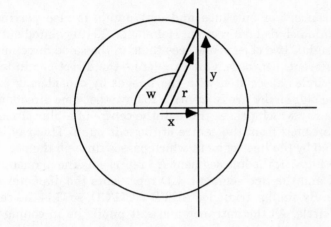

FIG. 5.4 Variables involved in calculation of the retinal light distribution

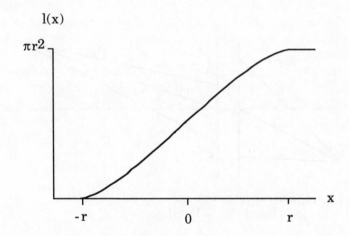

FIG. 5.5 Retinal luminance distribution associated with a step edge.

The variable x specifies retinal position with respect to an origin located at the image of the step in the plane of the retina and l(x) is the luminance level associated with the position x. The radius of the blur circle is r.

Angular Magnification

The concept of entrance and exit pupils is also pertinent to the definition of visual direction. Helmholtz (1910) pointed out that when one 'sights' two objects one sees them in the same direction, although at different distances. One can define the directions in terms of the blur circles associated with the images by considering two images, whose blur circles are concentric, to have the same direction.

The ray which passes through the centre of a blur circle is the ray which comes from the centre of the exit pupil. This ray is shown in Fig. 5.6 by the line segment which passes through the points F and G. As in Fig. 5.1, the line segment AB represents the diameter of the exit pupil and the line segment CD represents the diameter of the blur circle. By similar triangles AF/FB = CG/GD, so G is the centre of the blur circle. As the entrance and exit pupils lie in conjugate planes, any ray which hits the centre of the entrance pupil will emerge from the centre of the exit pupil. So each of the lines radiating from the centre of the entrance pupil specifies a DIRECTION LINE.

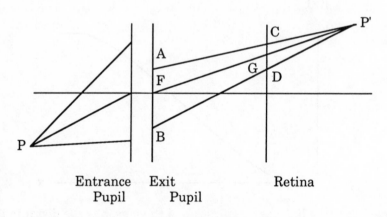

Entrance   Exit   Retina
Pupil   Pupil

FIG. 5.6. Ray through the centre of the blur circle

Since the entrance and exit pupils are conjugate planes, one can form the object - image transformation matrix and calculate the linear magnification between the planes. Direction lines can be represented by rays of the form [na, 0], which pass through the centre of the entrance pupil. It follows from the definition of the object - image transformation matrix that:

$$n'a' = na \,/\, m$$

so that the angular magnification carried out by the eyes is:

$$\frac{a'}{a} = \frac{n}{n'm}$$

For the human eye the value of the magnification factor is 0.813, so that a point 1 degree out in the visual field will be imaged 0.813 degrees out in the eye. Since the focal point of the eye lies 20.54 millimetres behind the exit pupil, this angle corresponds to a distance of approximately 0.3 millimetres in the focal plane. Thus 0.3 millimetres on the retina, corresponds to a visual angle of approximately 1 degree.

The angular magnification which results from placing a lens before the eye, can best be understood by breaking down the angular magnification into three constituent components. This approach follows that of Ogle (1950).

The first component relates to the power of the lens. The geometry involved is shown in Fig. 5.7, where it has been assumed that the distance between the entrance and exit pupils is negligible. In the paraxial case, the angular magnification μ produced by the lens can be formulated as follows:

$$\mu = \frac{a'}{a} \approx \frac{\tan a'}{\tan a} = \frac{\dfrac{h'}{y}}{\dfrac{h}{x}} = \frac{mx}{y}$$

where m is the linear magnification of the lens, x is the distance from the entrance pupil to the object plane and y is the distance from the entrance pupil to the image plane.

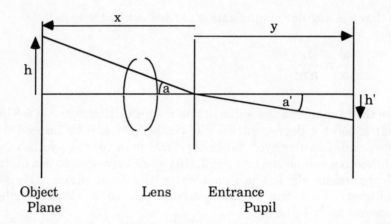

Object   Lens   Entrance
Plane   Pupil

FIG. 5.7. Geometry of angular magnification produced by a power
lens

In order to be able to use the expressions for m, derived in the
previous chapter, one has to introduce the reduced distances to the
object and image planes with respect to the lens vertices, shown in
Fig. 5.8. As the lens is in air, the reduced distances are equal to the
actual distances.

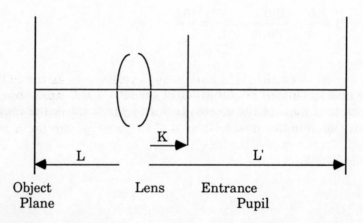

Object   Lens   Entrance
Plane   Pupil

FIG. 5.8. Distances used in calculation of the magnification of the lens

The analysis is simplified by considering a 'thin' lens in which the distance between the front and back surfaces of the lens is negligible. The system matrix of such a lens has the form:

$$S = \begin{bmatrix} 1 & -d \\ 0 & 1 \end{bmatrix}$$

where $d = d_1 + d_2$, which is the sum of the front and back surface powers. It follows from the conjugacy equations that the conjugacy relation for a thin lens in air is:

$$dLL' + L - L' = 0$$

and that the linear magnification $m = L'/L$. With this value, the equation describing the angular magnification caused by a lens becomes:

$$\mu = \frac{L'x}{L(L' - K)}$$

where K is the reduced distance between the posterior lens vertex and the entrance pupil. When the object is distant $x \approx L$ so:

$$\mu \approx \frac{1}{1 - \dfrac{K}{L'}}$$

The expression on the right hand side is referred to as the POWER factor and is denoted by the capital letter P. The factor is so-called because it is depends on the power of the lens when the object is distant, whereupon $d = 1/L'$ by definition of power for a single surface. In the case of a 'thick' lens $1/L'$ is referred to as the BACK VERTEX POWER of the lens.

If the distance K is taken to be 15 millimetres then a 1 dioptre power lens will result in approximately 1.5% of angular magnification. Spectacle wearers will be able to discern the effects of this angular magnification. Shortsightedness is corrected by minus lenses, which will reduce the angular extent of the image, while longsightedness is corrected by positive lenses which will increase the angular extent of the image.

The second component relates to the way in which the front and back surfaces of the lens act together like a simple telescope. In a telescopic system parallel rays entering the system emerge parallel, but at a changed orientation with respect to the optical axis. Since the change in the orientation of the ray is independent of the height of the ray above the optical axis, the element s_{12} of the system matrix of the lens must be zero. Hence, the system matrix for a single lens given in the previous chapter simplifies to:

$$S = \begin{bmatrix} 1 - d_2T & 0 \\ T & 1 - d_1T \end{bmatrix}$$

Hence n'a' = $(1-d_2T)$na and the angular magnification is $(1-d_2T)$. Since the determinant of the system matrix is unity:

$$\mu = 1 - d_2T = \frac{1}{1 - d_1T}$$

The term $1/(1 - d_1T)$ is referred to as the SHAPE FACTOR of the lens and is denoted by the capital letter S.

The final component relates to the way in which the lens acts like a plane glass plate. Since a plane surface has no power, the system matrix S (note the italics which signify a matrix rather than the shape factor) for a plane plate consists of a single translation matrix:

$$S = \begin{bmatrix} 1 & 0 \\ T & 1 \end{bmatrix}$$

and the associated matrix for the object to image transformation is equal to:

$$TST = \begin{bmatrix} 1 & 0 \\ L' + T - L & 1 \end{bmatrix}$$

hence L' - L = T. As L' is measured from the opposite side of the plate to L, it follows that the distance between the object and its image is equal to (1-1/n)t, where t is the thickness of the plate. The angular magnification caused by a plane plate is shown in Fig. 5.9. The object to image transformation matrix for the plate implies that the linear magnification m = 1, hence the sizes of the object h and its image h' are equal. Let the distance from the entrance pupil to the object be denoted by x, then the angular magnification is given by:

$$\mu = \frac{a'}{a} = \frac{\dfrac{h'}{x + (1 - \dfrac{1}{n})t}}{\dfrac{h}{x}} = \frac{1}{1 - (\dfrac{1}{n} - 1)\dfrac{t}{x}}$$

The term on the right hand side of this equation is referred to as the DISTANCE FACTOR and is denoted by Q.

In general, a lens will result in angular magnification involving all three of the factors; power P, shape S and distance Q. If these factors are independent, then the overall angular magnification of a lens will be given by their product PSQ. That this is true will be demonstrated in the next section.

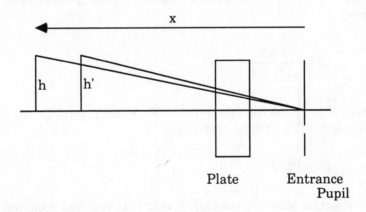

FIG. 5.9. Angular magnification caused by a plane plate

Combination of Angular Magnifications

The formal derivation of the angular magnification factors follows that of Ogle (1936) and is something of a slog; the derivation is included mainly for reference. Using the distances shown in Fig. 5.8, the equation for angular magnification due to a lens becomes:

$$\mu = \frac{mx}{L' - K}$$

The linear magnification m can be expressed in terms of the distances to the object and image planes by applying the conjugacy equations:

$$\mu = \frac{L'x}{(-s_{21} + s_{22})(L' - K)}$$

Substituting the values for s_{21} and s_{22} corresponding to the system matrix of a single lens, as derived in chapter 4:

$$\mu = \frac{L'x}{(-T + (1 - d_1T)L)(L' - K)} = \frac{Px}{-T + (1 - d_1T)L}$$

where $P = 1/(1-K/L')$ is the power factor. Dividing through by $(1-d_1T)$ gives

$$\mu = \frac{PSx}{-TS + L}$$

where S is the shape factor $1/(1-d_1T)$. Finally, letting the distance factor $Q = x / (L - TS)$ one can write:

$$\mu = PSQ$$

For a single lens the conjugacy relations can be expanded out by substituting for values from the system matrix:

$$\frac{1}{L'} = \frac{s_{11} + s_{12}}{s_{21} + s_{22}}\frac{L}{L} = \frac{(1 - d_2T) + (d_1 + d_2 - d_1d_2T)L}{-T + (1 - d_1T)L}$$

and if the terms equal to the shape factor are represented by S

$$= \frac{(1 - d_2T) + (\dfrac{d_2}{S} + d_1)L}{-T + \dfrac{L}{S}} = \frac{(1 - d_2T)S + VL}{L - TS}$$

where the back vertex power of the lens $V = Sd_1 + d_2$, since when L is large $1/L' = V$. The expression for $1/L'$ can be further simplified by factoring the numerator:

$$\frac{1}{L'} = \frac{(1 - d_2T)S + S^2d_1T + d_2TS + V(L - TS)}{L - TS}$$

$$= V + \frac{S(1 + Sd_1T)}{L - TS} = V + \frac{S(\dfrac{1 - d_1T + d_1T}{1 - d_1T})}{L - TS}$$

$$= V + \frac{S^2}{L - TS}$$

With the formulation of $1/L'$ given in this equation, the power and distance factors can be redefined to make their meaning relate directly to the different optical techniques for producing angular magnification of the image.

$$PSQ = \frac{SQ}{1 - VK - \dfrac{S^2K}{L - ST}} = \frac{P'SQ}{1 - \dfrac{P'S^2K}{L - ST}}$$

where P' = 1 / (1-VK). This form of the power factor gives the magnification caused by the power of a lens when the object is distant. The alternative form for the distance factor is derived by rearranging the equation:

$$PSQ = \frac{P'Sx}{(L - ST) - P'S^2K} = \frac{P'Sx}{(x + K + t - ST) - P'S^2K}$$

$$= \frac{P'Sx}{x + (1 - P'S^2)K - (S - n)T} = P'SQ'$$

where Q' = x / (x + (1 - P'S^2)K - (S-n)T). When the lens has no curvature S = 1 and P = 1 and this form of the distance factor becomes:

$$Q' = \frac{1}{1 - (1 - n)\dfrac{T}{x}}$$

which is the magnification produced by a plane glass plate.

Summary

The entrance pupil is the object which is imaged onto the actual pupil by the cornea. The exit pupil is the image of the actual pupil which is formed by the lens. In the human eye the entrance and exit pupils lie 3.04 and 3.68 millimetres respectively, behind the anterior vertex of the cornea.

If the image of a point is not formed in the plane of the retina, then it will consist of a blur circle whose diameter is proportional to the diameter of the exit pupil. Let f' and x' be the positions of the focal point and the image point, both specified with respect to the exit pupil. If e denotes the diameter of the exit pupil, then the diameter b of the blur circle is given by the formula:

$$b = \frac{ex'}{f' + x'}$$

The line from the centre of the entrance pupil to an object point specifies the direction of the point. As well as altering the sizes of the blur circles, the effect of placing an optical system in front of the eye will be to change the directions of the lines radiating from the centre of the entrance pupil, resulting in angular magnification of the image.

When an object is distant, the angular magnification produced by a lens, with a front surface power of d_1 and a back surface power of d_2, will depend on the product of its shape factor S:

$$S = \frac{1}{1 - d_1 T}$$

and its power factor P:

$$P = \frac{1}{1 - VK}$$

where V is the back vertex power of the lens, which is equal to $Sd_1 + d_2$, and K is the distance from the lens to the eye.

CHAPTER 6

Binocular Vision

Angular magnification does not cause a problem when viewing with only one eye, because objects simply look nearer. However, when both eyes are involved angular magnifications can lead to apparent distortions of objects. It was Wheatstone (1838) who first appreciated that the separation of the eyes results in each eye forming a slightly different image of the scene, and investigated the role of these slight differences by presenting planar projections of objects to each eye, rather than the objects themselves. In the Wheatstone stereoscope when separate pictures of a scene, which differ only in vantage point, are delivered to each eye then the scene appears three - dimensional. The distortions in stereovision which are caused by angular magnification of the image in one eye are analysed in this chapter.

Components of Disparities

The stimulus for stereoscopic vision can be specified in terms of the directions associated with the retinal images in the two eyes. Each point in the scene has an associated DISPARITY, which is given by the difference between the direction of the image of the point in the left eye and the direction of the image of the point in the right eye. The relationship between the position of a point in space and its disparity can be appreciated by considering the locus of points, referred to as the HOROPTER, which have the same direction in each eye and so have zero disparity. The simplest form of the horopter is associated with points on a plane which passes through the point of fixation and the centres of the entrance pupils of the two eyes. In this case the points on the horopter form a circle, referred to as the Vieth - Müller circle.

If the line from the centre of the entrance pupil of the left eye to the point of fixation F is taken to be the zero direction in that eye, then the direction of any point P is specified by the angle x_l, which is made by the line from the centre of the entrance pupil to the point P and the zero direction. The corresponding angle in the right eye is x_r, as shown in Fig. 6.1. The disparity associated with any point P can then be defined to be equal to the difference $x_l - x_r$ between the directions in the left and right eyes.

It follows from Euclidean geometry that all the points on the Veith - Müller circle have zero disparity. The disparities associated with points beyond the Vieth - Müller circle are referred to as uncrossed, and the disparities associated with points inside the circle are referred to as crossed, in keeping with the uncrossed and crossed diplopia that arises when these disparities are large.

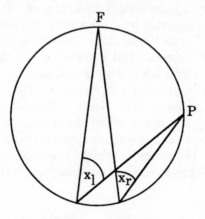

Left Eye   Right Eye

FIG. 6.1. Variables used in defining the disparity of a point P. The Vieth - Müller circle delineates the locus of point with zero disparity.

The drawback of this geometric approach to understanding disparity is that when the restriction to points in a plane is lifted, then it is not always possible to find points with zero disparity. However, Mayhew (1982) devised an alternative framework for describing the disparities associated with objects which do not lie in the horizontal plane. He distinguished between horizontal and vertical disparities because they vary differently from each other, and was able to show that the horizontal disparity H is comprised of three components and that the vertical disparity V is comprised of two components. The components of horizontal disparity are H_{depth} - the disparity due to depth, H_{gaze} - the disparity due to gaze angle and $H_{eccentricity}$ - the disparity due to eccentricity in the visual field. The components of vertical disparity are V_{gaze} and $V_{eccentricity}$ - due to gaze angle and eccentricity respectively.

The variables used in his analysis are shown in Fig. 6.2. The distance between the two eyes is denoted by s. The location of the point of fixation F is specified in terms of two parameters, both of which are specified with respect to the entrance pupil of the cyclopean eye. The gaze angle g is equal to the angle that the line of sight of a cyclopean eye makes with the point of fixation. The distance parameter d specifies how far along this direction the point of fixation is. The direction of the point of fixation gives the depth axis and the depth equals 0 for all points lying on the plane which is normal to the the depth direction and passes through the point of fixation. The depth of a point P is denoted by z.

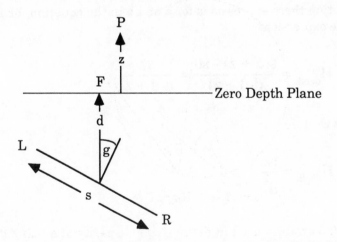

FIG. 6.2. Variables used in the analysis of disparity. s is the separation between the left eye (L) and the right eye (R). d is the distance to the point of fixation (F), and g is the angle which specifies the direction of the point of fixation. z is the distance, relative to the point of fixation, to the point P.

The component H_{depth} of horizontal disparity due to depth can be determined by considering the case of a point P lying behind the point of fixation when the eyes are symmetrically converged by an angle of 2a. This situation is shown in Fig. 6.3. If the angle of convergence at the point P is 2b then

$$H_{depth} = 2(a - b)$$

If the angles a and b are small they can be expressed in terms of the interocular separation s and the distance to the point of fixation d:

$$a = \frac{s}{2d}$$

and

$$b = \frac{s}{2(d + z)}$$

substituting these expressions for a and b in the equation for H_{depth} gives the expression:

$$H_{depth} = \frac{s(d + z) - sd}{d(d + z)} = \frac{sz}{d(d + z)}$$

and as z « d

$$H_{depth} = \frac{sz}{d^2}$$

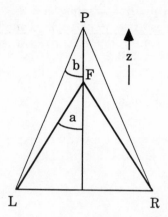

FIG. 6.3. Calculation of the horizontal disparities due to depth

If the angles x and x' are the horizontal eccentricities of the point P in the left and right eyes respectively then the horizontal disparity H_{gaze} due to gaze angle is equal to:

$$H_{gaze} = x - x'$$

and if x and x' are small:

$$H_{gaze} = \frac{PF}{PL} - \frac{PF}{PR} = x(1 - \frac{PL}{PR})$$

An approximation to the ratio PL / PR can be made in terms of the distance to the point of fixation d , the interocular separation s and the gaze angle g as shown in Fig. 6.4. Using this approximation, the equation for H_{gaze} becomes:

$$H_{gaze} = x\left(1 - \frac{d - \frac{s}{2} \sin g}{d + \frac{s}{2} \sin g}\right)$$

$$= x\left(\frac{d + \frac{s}{2}\sin g - d + \frac{s}{2}\sin g}{d + \frac{s}{2}\sin g}\right) = \frac{s \sin g\ x}{d + \frac{s}{2}\sin g}$$

and since g is small and s/2 sin g « d

$$H_{gaze} \approx \frac{sgx}{d}$$

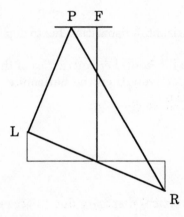

FIG. 6.4. Approximation to the ratio PL / PR

The horizontal disparity $H_{eccentricity}$ due to eccentricity is the same as that involved if the eyes turn through the gaze angle g to fixate a point and so:

$$H_{eccentricity} \approx \frac{sx^2}{d}$$

Vertical disparity arises when a point is nearer to one eye than to the other. The vertical disparity due to gaze angle can be obtained by considering a point whose images lie on the vertical meridians of each eye, and proceeding as with horizontal disparity. Let y and y' be the vertical eccentricities in the left and right eyes respectively of a point directly above the point of fixation, then:

$$V_{gaze} = y - y'$$

and if y and y' are small then:

$$V_{gaze} = \frac{PF}{PL} - \frac{PF}{PR} = y(1 - \frac{PL}{PR})$$

Again the ratio of PL / PR can be approximated in terms of s, d and g:

$$V_{gaze} = y\left(1 - \frac{d - \frac{s}{2} \sin g}{d + \frac{s}{2} \sin g}\right) = \frac{s \sin g \, y}{d + \frac{s}{2} \sin g}$$

and as before, since g is small and s/2 sin g « d

$$V_{gaze} \approx \frac{sgy}{d}$$

Similarly, the component of vertical disparity due to eccentricity is given by:

$$V_{eccentricity} \approx \frac{sxy}{d}$$

Motion and Stereoscopic Parallax

A general framework for analysing stereoscopic vision is provided by considering it as an instance of the change of view that is associated with change in the position of the eyes. Longuet-Higgins and Prazdny (1980) analysed the geometry of parallax with a moving observer by applying the approach of classical mechanics, in which the motion of a rigid body is described in terms of the individual particles which make up the body. In their formulation, each point in the scene corresponds to a vector **p** in a right handed system of Cartesian base vectors which are located at the centre of the entrance pupil and are fixed with respect to the eye so that the **e₃** direction points away from the retina as shown in Fig. 6.5.

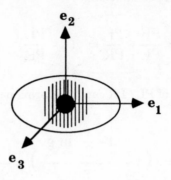

FIG. 6.5. Right handed system of Cartesian base vectors, fixed with respect to the centre of the entrance pupil

If the eye of the observer moves with a velocity **v** then:

$$\frac{d\mathbf{p}}{dt} = -\mathbf{v}$$

The eye can also change its orientation by rotating in its socket. In general, if **r** is a point on a body which is rotating about an axis lying in the direction **w**, with an angular velocity of w radians per second, then the point will move around a circular path as shown in Fig. 6.6. The radius of the circular path is |**r**| sin q, and the instantaneous rate of change of position is w |**r**| sin q. Since the direction of the change of position is perpendicular to the plane spanned by **w** and **r**, one can set the length of **w** equal to w and then:

$$\frac{d\mathbf{r}}{dt} = \mathbf{w}^{\wedge}\mathbf{r}$$

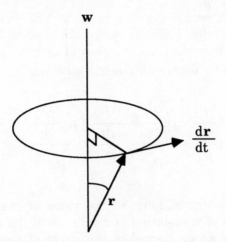

FIG. 6.6. Calculation of the angular velocity of a point on a rotating body

Hence, if the eye of an observer rotates about an axis **w** with angular velocity |**w**| then:

$$\frac{d\mathbf{p}}{dt} = - \mathbf{w}^\wedge \mathbf{p}$$

Combining the effects of the translation and rotation of the eye of the observer gives an expression for dp/dt which can be expanded out in terms of coordinates:

$$\frac{d\mathbf{p}}{dt} =$$

$$(-v_1 - w_2 p_3 + w_3 p_2 \, , \, -v_2 + w_1 p_3 - w_3 p_1 \, , \, -v_3 - w_1 p_2 + w_2 p_1 \,)$$

The planar projection of the retinal image (x,y) can be obtained by considering the projection of the point specified by **p** into a plane at unit distance in the direction of the e_3 base vector.

$$(x, y) = (\frac{p_1}{p_3}, \frac{p_2}{p_3})$$

Applying the formula for differentiation of a quotient:

$$(\frac{dx}{dt}, \frac{dy}{dt}) = (\frac{\frac{dp_1}{dt}}{p_3} - \frac{p_1 \frac{dp_3}{dt}}{p_3^2}, \frac{\frac{dp_2}{dt}}{p_3} - \frac{p_2 \frac{dp_3}{dt}}{p_3^2})$$

and substituting the expressions for the rates of change of the coordinates in terms of translation and rotation of the eye gives a general formulation which describes the effect of motion of the observer on the retinal image:

$$\frac{dx}{dt} = -\frac{v_1}{p_3} - w_2 + w_3\, y + \frac{v_3\, x}{p_3} + w_1\, xy - w_2\, x^2$$

$$= \frac{-v_1 + v_3\, x}{p_3} + w_1\, xy - (1 + x^2)w_2 + w_3\, y$$

and

$$\frac{dy}{dt} = -\frac{v_2}{p_3} + w_1 - w_3\, x + \frac{v_3\, y}{p_3} + w_1\, y^2 - w_2\, xy$$

$$= \frac{-v_2 + v_3\, y}{p_3} + (1 + y^2)w_1 - w_2\, xy - w_3\, x$$

The geometry of stereovision is equivalent to the geometry of vision with a moving eye, except that the retinal image is differentiated with respect to a spatial variable t, rather than with respect to time. By analogy with the moving eye case, an eye can be asssumed to move from the position of the right eye to the position of the left. The movement of the eye involves a translation in the e_1e_3 plane described by the vector **v**, and an anticlockwise rotation about the e_2 direction described by the vector **w**. When g is small:

$$\mathbf{v} = (s, 0, sg)$$

and

$$\mathbf{w} = (0, -\frac{s}{d}, 0)$$

where s is the interocular separation and d is the distance to the point of fixation, as in the previous section. As before, let z be the depth relative to the point of fixation, then:

$$(\frac{dx}{dt}, \frac{dy}{dt}) = (\frac{-s + sgx}{d + z} + \frac{s(1 + x^2)}{d}, \frac{sgy}{d + z} + \frac{sxy}{d})$$

$$= (\frac{-sd + sdgx + s(d + z)}{d(d + z)} + \frac{sx^2}{d}, \frac{sgy}{d + z} + \frac{sxy}{d})$$

and as z « d

$$(\frac{dx}{dt}, \frac{dy}{dt}) \approx \frac{s}{d}(\frac{z}{d} + gx + x^2, gy + xy)$$

The terms on the right hand side of this equation are identical to the components of disparity isolated by Mayhew's analysis. The two different approaches to deriving these equations are similar to the two different approaches used to derive the equations for the angular magnification caused by a lens. In the intuitive approach, the individual components are analysed on their own, and the relationship between them is guessed at. In the formal approach the components drop out as terms in the equations. The derivations of the factors involved in angular magnification by a lens, and of the factors involved in generating disparities, illustrate the point that whilst a phenomenon can be analysed by breaking it down into its component parts, understanding the relationship between the parts usually requires a general theoretical framework.

Patterns of Disparities

The formal description of stereoscopic parallax can be thought of as capturing the differences between the images of the left and right eyes, as seen by the cyclopean eye. The resulting pattern of disparities can be understood by drawing the image of the right eye and overplotting the image of the left eye. The simplest patterns of disparities are associated with points lying on a plane perpendicular to the gaze direction which passes through the point of fixation. Such a plane will be referred to as a frontal plane. Let the gaze angle be zero, and let the stimulus consist of the central 10 degree by 10 degree square of a frontal plane, then the forms of the overplotted images of the outline of the square are as shown in Fig. 6.7. The image in the right eye is shown in bold.

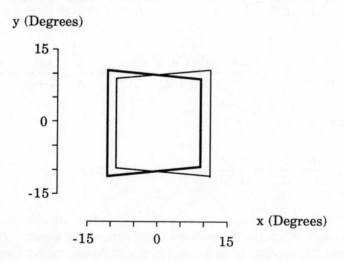

FIG. 6.7. Exaggerated differences between the images of a square in the right and left eyes. The thick line represents the image in the right eye.

It is clear from the geometric representation of the two images that one can associate a plane vector with each point in the image of the right eye, which translates the point to the corresponding point in the image of the left eye. If one plots the disparity vectors associated with a regularly spaced array of points in the frontal plane, when the gaze angle is zero, then one obtains the characteristic radial pattern of disparities shown in Fig. 6.8. As is usual with disparities, the easiest to comprehend are those associated with points lying in the plane of the Vieth - Müller circle. Since the frontal plane lies beyond the circle, except at the point of fixation, the disparities associated with the points are all uncrossed, so the image in the left eye always appears to the left of the image in the right eye, in the cyclopean eye. In the right handed system of base vectors being used in this analysis, being on the left corresponds to a positive x value.

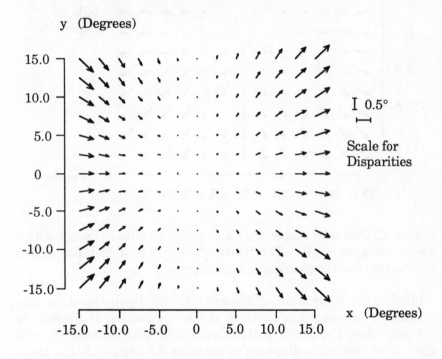

Figure 6.8 Disparities associated with eccentricity of points on a frontal plane. The fixation point is at a distance of 573 millimetres and the gaze angle is zero.

One can similarly plot the disparity vectors associated with the component of disparity due to gaze angle, as has been done in Fig. 6.9 for a 15 degree gaze angle. The right half of the frontal plane lies beyond the Vieth - Müller circle and so the pattern of disparities has the same form as that due to eccentricity. However, the left half of the frontal plane lies inside the horopter circle, and so the pattern of disparities is reversed for the left half.

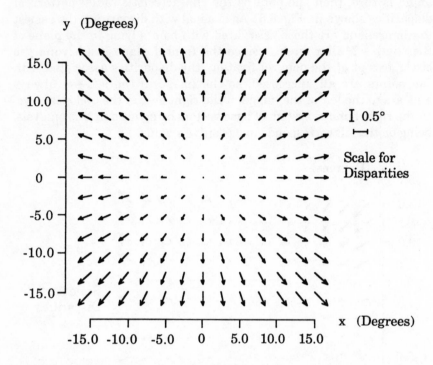

Figure 6.9 Disparities associated with points on a frontal plane with a 15 degree gaze angle. The fixation point is at a distance of 573 millimetres and the gaze angle is 15 degrees.

Finally, the component of disparity due to depth involves only horizontal differences in direction and so the pattern of disparity is different from the radial pattern associated with eccentricity and gaze. The horizontal disparity is the same for any point on a plane parallel to the frontal plane, as shown in figure 6.10. This example was generated by considering points on a fronto - parallel plane which lay 40 millimetres beyond the point of fixation.

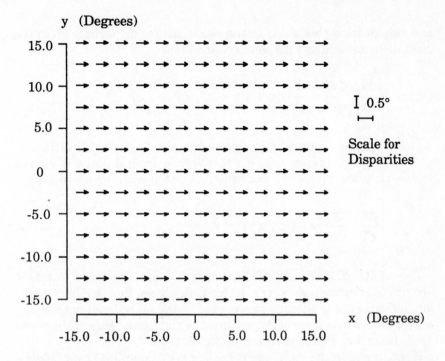

Figure 6.10 Disparities associated with points on a plane parallel to the frontal plane but lying 40 millimetres beyond the point of fixation. The fixation point is at a distance of 573 millimetres and the gaze angle is 0 degrees.

The visual system is able to separate out the pattern of disparity due to depth from the extraneous patterns due to eccentricity and gaze angle. The evidence for this finding comes from the effects of meridional magnifying lenses which were analysed by Mayhew and Longuet - Higgins (1982). Their analytical techniques will be used in the treatment given here.

The equation of a vertical plane through the point of fixation is:

$$p_3 = cp_1 + d$$

where c is a constant which specifies the slope of the plane. Since $z = p_3 - d$ it follows that:

$$z = cp_1$$

and substituting this value in the equations for disparities gives the disparities associated with points on the plane:

$$(\frac{dx}{dt}, \frac{dy}{dt}) \approx \frac{s}{d}(cx + gx + x^2, gy + xy)$$

A frontal plane is one which is perpendicular to the e_3 direction, as shown in Fig. 6.11a, so that $c = 0$. When a frontal plane is viewed with symmetric gaze, the disparities associated with the plane are:

$$(\frac{dx}{dt}, \frac{dy}{dt}) \approx \frac{s}{d}(x^2, xy)$$

The GEOMETRIC EFFECT refers to the apparent rotation around a vertical axis of a frontal plane due to horizontal magnification of the image in one eye. If the meridional magnifying lens is placed over the right eye, then the right hand side of the plane appears further away, as shown in Fig. 6.11b.

If the image in the right eye is horizontally magnified by a factor h then the disparities associated with the image of the frontal plane have an additional component which is independent of the distance to the point of fixation and the separation of the eyes:

$$(\frac{dx}{dt}, \frac{dy}{dt}) \approx \frac{s}{d}((1 - h)\frac{dx}{s} + x^2, xy)$$

which is equivalent to the disparities associated with points on a vertical plane which is slanted so that:

$$c = (1 - h)\frac{d}{s}$$

since $s \ll d$.

The INDUCED EFFECT refers to the apparent rotation around a vertical axis of a frontal plane due to vertical magnification of the image in one eye. If the meridional magnifying lens is placed over the right eye, then the right hand side of the plane appears nearer, as shown in Fig. 6.11c. If the image of the right eye is vertically magnified by a factor v then the disparities associated with the image of the frontal plane become:

$$(\frac{dx}{dt}, \frac{dy}{dt}) \approx \frac{s}{d} (x^2, (1 - v)\frac{dy}{s} + xy)$$

which is equivalent to the disparity present in a slanted plane when the gaze angle is equal to (1 - v)d/s. If one assumes that the gaze angle is (1 - v)d/s, then the pattern of disparites is equal to that of a frontal plane slanted in the opposite direction to the geometrically produced slant:

$$(\frac{dx}{dt}, \frac{dy}{dt}) \approx (- (1 - v)\frac{dx}{s} + (1 - v)\frac{dx}{s} + x^2, (1 - v)\frac{dy}{s} + xy)$$

The slant of this plane is such that:

$$c = - (1 - v)\frac{d}{s}$$

so that for a given magnification the slant due to vertical magnification of one image is equal and opposite to that due to a horizontal magnification.

It is not surprising that the disparities associated with vertical magnification of one image are equal to a set of disparities obtained with a non - zero gaze angle. If one considers points on a vertical line passing through the point of fixation (for which x = 0) then it follows from Mayhew's geometrical analysis that the vertical disparities of these points, caused by vertical magnification of one image, can only occur naturally with a non zero gaze angle. Since g = (1-v)d/s, the gaze angle depends on the distance to the point of fixation. Putting s = 65 millimetres and d = 400 millimetres one obtains g = - 8.8 degrees for a magnification of 2.5%. But when d = 2000 millimetres, the predicted gaze angle is - 44 degrees. As pointed out by Mayhew and Longuet - Higgins (1982), since such a gaze angle could not occur in reality, it is unreasonable to expect the nervous system to have developed the capability of processing such disparities, and the induced effect is not reported with such stimulus arrangements.

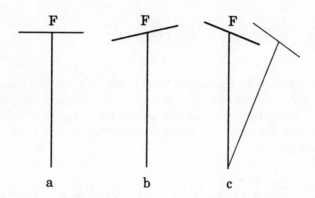

FIG. 6.11. Apparent positions of a frontal plane with a) no magnification, b) horizontal magnification and c) vertical magnification of the image of the right eye. The thin line shows the gaze direction stimulus plane which would gives rise to the same pattern of disparities as that of a frontal plane when the image in one eye is vertically magnified.

Why is the induced effect surprising? Because after vertical magnification of the image in one eye the two retinal images cannot possibly have come from a physical object - and one would expect to see double images. The geometric analysis shows that the two images can come from a physical object - but only if the eyes are assumed to be asymmetrically converged rather than in the positions which they are actually in. The implication of the induced effect is that the nervous system is able to separate the depth disparity pattern from the patterns of disparity due to eccentricity in the visual field and gaze angle. How it does this is an open question.

Example Calculation: Disparity fields associated with a plane surface

Load the PlotField.m package in Mathematica. The command will be of the form:

<< PlotField.m

but the specification of the path to the PlotField file will depend on the implementation of Mathematica on your system. To obtain a plot of the disparity field associated with a frontal plane, with x and y varying from -15 to +15 degrees in steps of 5 degrees, type in:

PlotVectorField[{(65/573)*(x^2), (65/573)*(x*y)},
            {x, -15.0/57.3, 15.0/57.3, 5/57.3},
            {y, -15.0/57.3, 15.0/57.3, 5/57.3}]

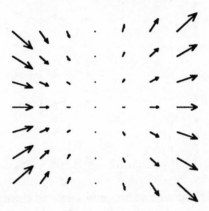

The effect of vertical magnification of the image in the right eye by 2.5% can be investigated by changing the command to:

PlotVectorField[{(65/573)*(x^2), -0.025*y + (65/573)*(x*y)},
            {x, -15.0/57.3, 15.0/57.3, 5/57.3},
            {y, -15.0/57.3, 15.0/57.3, 5/57.3}]

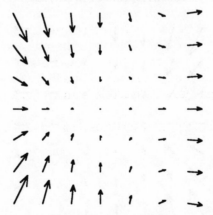

For comparison, the next two plots lead to the disparity field associated with a slanted plane viewed with asymmetric gaze. First calculate the disparity field associated with the slanted plane:

PlotVectorField[{0.025*x + (65/573)*(x^2), (65/573)*(x*y)},
            {x, -15.0/57.3, 15.0/57.3, 5/57.3},
            {y, -15.0/57.3, 15.0/57.3, 5/57.3}]

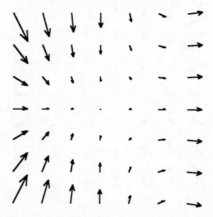

Secondly, plot the field when the gaze angle is changed to be equal to the negative of the slant of the plane. As can be seen, the disparity field plot is identical to that obtained with vertical magnification of the image in the right eye.

PlotVectorField[{0.025*x + (65/573)*(-0.025*(573/65)*x +x^2),
            (65/573)*(-0.025*(573/65)*y + x*y)},
            {x, -15.0/57.3, 15.0/57.3, 5/57.3},
            {y, -15.0/57.3, 15.0/57.3, 5/57.3}]

Summary

The disparity of a point is the difference between the directions of the images of the point in the left and right eyes. If the position of the point is described in a right handed system of Cartesian base vectors, with its origin at the centre of the entrance pupil of the cyclopean eye, then the horizontal disparity H of the point is given by the function:

$$H = \frac{s}{d} \left(\frac{z}{d} + gx + x^2 \right)$$

and the vertical disparity V of the point is given by the function:

$$V = \frac{s}{d} \left(gy + xy \right)$$

where s is the interocular distance, d is the distance to the point of fixation, g is the gaze angle of the eyes and x and y are the retinal directions of the point in the cyclopean eye.

CHAPTER 7

Neural Coding

In this chapter a framework is developed for investigating the stimulus patterns represented in neural mechanisms. An analysis of linear model neurons is used to obtain the simplest description of the patterns represented by a neural mechanism and this approach is applied in the subsequent chapters to reveal the aspects of the stimulus which are being captured by the colour and spatial coding mechanisms.

Hebbian Learning

The formalism of matrix algebra can be thought of as describing the behaviour of some form of machine, which has n inputs and m outputs. Corresponding to the matrix equation

$$y = Ax$$

one can envisage a machine with n inputs x_1, x_2, ...x_n whose levels are described by the vector x, and m outputs y_1, y_2, ...y_m whose levels are described by the vector y. Whenever the machine is presented with a set of inputs x it produces the set of outputs y, as specified by the m x n matrix A.

What might be the mechanism of such a machine? One can use the matrix description of the behaviour of the machine to break up its mechanism into simple computing elements referred to as LINEAR

FILTERS. Each linear filter has n inputs x_1, x_2, ... x_n and one output y. Associated with each input x_j is a 'weight', w_j and the function which associates a weight with each input is referred to as the WEIGHTING FUNCTION. The contribution of an input to the output of the filter is given by the level of the input multiplied by its weight, and the overall output of the filter is equal to the sum of the weighted inputs w_1x_1, w_2x_2,...w_nx_n. In formal notation the output is given by:

$$y = \sum_{j=1}^{n} w_j x_j = w^T x$$

Linear filters can be thought of as simple models of neurons, especially if they are drawn as shown in Fig. 7.1. The weighted inputs w_1x_1, w_2x_2,...w_nx_n correspond to nerve fibres synapsing on the cell body, and the output y corresponds to the firing pattern recorded from the axon of the cell. In a more complete model, the output would be some threshold function of the sum of the weighted inputs. All such model neurons are referred to by the generic label of FORMAL NEURONS, to distinguish them from real neurons. Any collection of formal neurons is referred to as a NEURAL NETWORK.

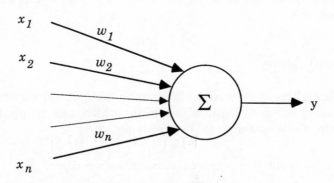

FIG 7.1 Pictorial representation of a linear filter

The range of behaviour of a neural network can be extended by assigning a learning rule to the neurons in the network. A simple form of learning is encapsulated in the HEBBIAN LEARNING RULE, which states that the weight associated with an input fibre of a neuron increases if the input fibre and the output fibre are active together. If the change in weight w_j associated with an input x_j is denoted by Δw_j, then the Hebbian rule can be described by the equation:

$$\Delta w_j = \eta x_j y$$

where η is a learning rate factor.

As it stands, the Hebbian rule leads to unstable behaviour in a neural net, because the weights can grow infinitely large. One way of ensuring stability with the Hebbian learning rule is to scale the weights so that the length of the weight vector is always equal to unity. If $w[t]$ denotes the weight vector at time t, the scaled changes in the weight vector are described by the equation:

$$w_j[t+1] = \frac{w_j[t] + \eta x_j[t]y[t]}{|(w[t] + \eta x[t]y[t])|}$$

This version of the Hebbian learning rule was developed by Oja (1982), who simplified it by using a linear approximation to the length of the weight vector.

The partial derivative of the length of the weight vector, with respect to the learning rate factor, can be evaluated by applying the chain rule for differentiation:

$$\frac{\partial \sqrt{\sum_{j=1}^{n}(w_j[t] + \eta x_j[t]y[t])^2}}{\partial \eta} =$$

$$\frac{\sum_{j=1}^{n}(w_j[t]x_j[t]y[t] + \eta x_j[t]^2 y[t]}{\sqrt{\sum_{j=1}^{n}(w_j[t] + \eta x_j[t]y[t])^2}}$$

Since the learning rate factor is assumed to be small, this partial derivative is evaluated at $\eta = 0$:

$$\frac{\partial \sqrt{\sum_{j=1}^{n} (w_j[t] + \eta x_j[t]y[t])^2}}{\partial \eta} \Bigg|_{\eta=0} =$$

$$\sum_{j=1}^{n} w_j[t] \, x_j[t]y[t] = y[t]^2$$

The length of the weight vector is equal to unity plus the small change in length which can be approximated by the partial derivative multiplied by the learning rate factor. Using this approximation, Oja's learning rule becomes:

$$w_j[t+1] \approx \frac{w_j[t] + \eta x_j[t]y[t]}{1 + \eta y[t]^2}$$

from which it follows that:

$$w_j[t+1] - w_j[t] = \eta x_j[t]y[t] - w_j[t+1]\eta y[t]^2$$

$$= \eta x_j[t]y[t] - w_j[t]\eta y[t]^2$$

since the terms involving η^2 are small enough to ignore. Hence Oja's learning rule can be simplified to:

$$\Delta w_j = \eta y(x_j - yw_j)$$

As an example of how this rule works in practice, consider a two input linear filter. Let the inputs to this filter be chosen at random from the range $-1 < x_1 < 1$ and $-0.25 < x_2 < 0.25$. If the input values are plotted in Cartesian coordinates, as shown in Fig. 7.2, then the possible input values lie in a rectangular region of the plane. A similar plot for the weight values is given in Fig. 7.3, with the final weight values being marked by a graphical representation of a vector. The continuous line leading to the the vector represents the weight values which the filter adopts during training. The initial weight values were chosen at random, subject to the constraint that the weight vector is of unit length.

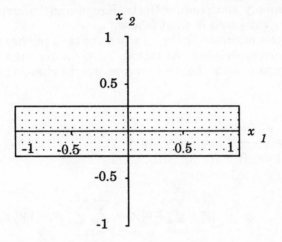

FIG. 7.2. Diagrammatic representation of the input values of a two input linear filter. The shaded region definess the range of inputs used in the example.

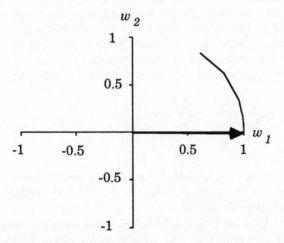

FIG. 7.3. Plot of the weight values during training. For the results shown in this figure, and in Figs. 7.5. and 7.6, the learning rate factor was 0.05, the training was stopped after 2500 input presentations, and the final weight values are marked by arrows.

Input Representation

Given a stable learning rule, one wants to know what is being learned by the linear filter. Hebbian learning rules have been comprehensively analysed by Hertz, Krogh and Palmer (1991), and their findings are used in what follows.

The analysis begins at the point when the training has resulted in a stable pattern of weights. At this stage in the training the average weight change is zero. Let the average weight change be denoted by $\langle \Delta w_j \rangle$, then:

$$0 = \langle \frac{\Delta w_j}{\eta} \rangle = \langle x_j y - w_j y^2 \rangle$$

$$= \langle \sum_{k=1}^{n} x_j w_k x_k - \sum_{l=1}^{n} \sum_{k=1}^{n} w_j w_l x_l w_k x_k \rangle$$

This average can be simplified by introducing the concept of a correlation between the inputs. The correlation between two inputs is a measure of how much the activity of the two inputs is related, and is computed simply by the product of the input values. If two inputs have values with the same sign, then there correlation is positive, whereas if the values are not of the same sign, then the correlation is negative. Let the CORRELATION MATRIX C be formed by the average of the correlations between each of the inputs i.e. $C_{ij} = \langle x_i x_j \rangle$, then the equilibrium equation becomes:

$$0 = \sum_{k=1}^{n} C_{kj} w_j - \sum_{l=1}^{n} \sum_{k=1}^{n} w_l C_{lk} w_k w_j = Cw - [w^T Cw]w$$

This equation is only satisfied if w is an eigenvector of C so that $Cw = \lambda w$. As the learning rule has been defined so that $|w| = 1$, it follows that $[w^T Cw]w = \lambda w$.

The final part of the analysis involves showing that the weight vector ends up equal to the largest eigenvector in the correlation matrix, scaled to unit length. Assume that the weight vector is close to a unit length eigenvector u:

$$w = u + \varepsilon$$

where the length of ε is much less than one. Substituting this formula for w in the equation for the average weight changes, and assuming that all terms involving $|\varepsilon|^2$ are negligibly small, gives the following equation for the average weight changes:

$$\langle \frac{\Delta w_j}{\eta} \rangle = C\,(u+\varepsilon) - [(u+\varepsilon)^T C\,(u+\varepsilon)](u+\varepsilon)$$

$$\approx \lambda u + C\varepsilon - [u^T Cu\,]u - [\varepsilon^T Cu\,]u - [u^T C\varepsilon]u - [u^T Cu\,]\varepsilon$$

After collecting like terms, the equation becomes:

$$\langle \frac{\Delta w_j}{\eta} \rangle = C\varepsilon - 2\lambda[\varepsilon^T u\,]u - \lambda\varepsilon$$

The key to the proof is to consider the projection of these average changes in the weight vector onto another unit length eigenvector v of the input correlation matrix. Let the eigenvalue associated with v be denoted by λ_v, then:

$$v^T \langle \frac{\Delta w_j}{\eta} \rangle = \lambda_v v^T \varepsilon - 2\lambda[\varepsilon^T u\,]v^T u - \lambda v^T \varepsilon$$

$$= (\lambda_v - \lambda - 2\lambda[v^T u\,]v^T \varepsilon$$

Except in the case when $u = v$, the scalar product $u\,.v$ will be zero as the eigenvectors are orthogonal. Hence if λ_v is greater than λ then the projection of the weight changes onto v will continue to grow. The average weight changes will only be stable when the weight vector lies in the direction of the eigenvector with the largest eigenvalue. In effect, the weight vector has become matched to the component of the input patterns which accounts for the largest part of the variation in the inputs.

In the case of the example given at the end of the last section the correlation matrix is:

$$C = \begin{bmatrix} 0.32 & 0 \\ 0 & 0.02 \end{bmatrix}$$

This matrix is already in diagonal form, and the largest eigenvalue can be read off as 0.32. The unit eigenvector associated with this eigenvalue is (1,0) and inspection of Fig.7.3 confirms that the weight vector converged to this eigenvector.

Eigenvector Transformation

Sanger (1989) extended Oja's learning rule to networks containing more than one output. If the m outputs are indexed by the variable i then Sanger's rule can be written as:

$$\Delta w_{ij} = \eta y_i \left(x_j - \sum_{k=1}^{i} y_k w_{kj} \right)$$

With this learning rule, the weights associated with successive neurons correspond to the successive eigenvectors of the input correlation matrix. The first output learns the eigenvector with the largest eigenvalue, the second output learns the eigenvector with the next largest eigenvalue and so on. Again following Hertz, Krogh and Palmer, one can prove this by considering the average weight changes after training:

$$0 = \langle \frac{\Delta w_{ij}}{\eta} \rangle = \langle x_j y_i - y_i \sum_{k=1}^{i} w_{kj} y_k \rangle$$

$$= \langle \sum_{l=1}^{n} x_j w_{il} x_l - \sum_{l=1}^{n} w_{il} x_l \sum_{k=1}^{i} w_{kj} \sum_{s=1}^{n} w_{ks} x_s \rangle$$

This equation is more complicated than that for a single neuron, because of the summation over the output neurons, but substitution of the correlation matrix leads to simplification of the equation, as before:

$$0 = \sum_{l=1}^{n} w_{il} C_{lj} - \sum_{k=1}^{i} \left[\sum_{l=1}^{n} \sum_{s=1}^{n} w_{ks} C_{ls} w_{il} \right] w_{kj}$$

and if the weight vector w_{i1}, $w_{i2} \dots w_{in}$ is denoted by ω_i then the right hand side of the equation can be written as:

$$= C\omega_i - \sum_{k=1}^{i} [\omega_k^T C\omega_l] \omega_k$$

The proof that the weights of successive outputs correspond to successive eigenvectors of the input correlation matrix makes use of the construction of a projection of one vector into a direction orthogonal to another vector. A graphical representation of this construction is shown in Fig. 7.4, from which it can be seen that if **x** is a vector and **y** is a unit vector, then the orthogonal projection of **x** onto **y** is equal to **x** - (**y**.**x**)**y**.

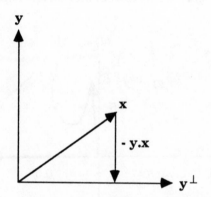

FIG. 7.4. Construction of the orthogonal projection of a vector **x** onto a unit vector **y**. The vector orthogonal to **y** is denoted by **y**⊥.

If one assumes that the weight vectors of the first i-1 outputs are equal to the first i-1 unit length eigenvectors, and can prove that the weight vector of the ith output is equal to the ith unit length eigenvector, then it is clear that this property holds for all outputs. Making use of the orthogonal projection construction, one can define the projection $(C\omega_i)^\perp$ of the ith weight vector multiplied by the input correlation matrix, onto a set of vectors orthogonal to the first i-1 eigenvectors. This projection is given by the formula:

$$(C\omega_i)^{\perp} = C\omega_i - \sum_{k=1}^{i-1} [\omega_i{}^{\mathrm{T}} C\omega_i]\omega_k$$

By applying this formula, the equation for the average weight changes with Sanger's learning rule can be rewritten as:

$$\langle \frac{\Delta\omega_i}{\eta} \rangle = (C\omega_i)^{\perp} - [\omega_i{}^{\mathrm{T}} C\omega_i]\omega_i$$

The weight vector ω_i will change until it becomes a linear combination of the set of vectors orthogonal to the first i-1 eigenvectors, but then the learning rule will act just like Oja's, and the weight vector will end up matching the largest eigenvector of $(C\omega_i)^{\perp}$, as required. Fig. 7.5. extends the example from one to two outputs. The first output learns the larger eigenvector, as before, and the second output learns the smaller eigenvector.

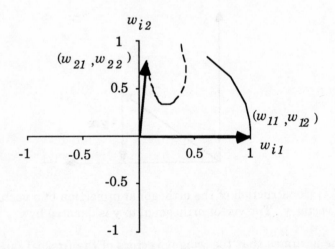

FIG. 7.5. Plot of the weight values for two outputs trained according to Sanger's rule.

Oja's own extension of his rule to a network containing more than one output neuron involves summation over all the outputs:

$$\Delta w_{ij} = \eta y_i \left(x_j - \sum_{k=1}^{m} y_k w_{kj} \right)$$

The weight vectors learned with this rule are all orthogonal, but they consist of linear combinations of the unit eigenvectors of the input correlation matrix, rather than individual eigenvectors on their own This result is apparent from the behaviour of the example network, trained according to Oja's learning rule, which is shown in Fig.7.6.

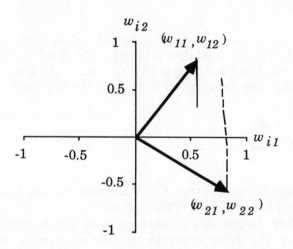

FIG. 7.6 Example of the changes in the weight vectors during training with Oja's learning rule.

In the context of developing a framework for interpreting neural coding, the differences between Oja's and Sanger's learning rules are very important. Irrespective of the biological validity of the two learning rules, what they show is that neural networks can code the same information in a variety of ways, some of which are easier to interpret than others. Oja's rule results in neurons which are more biologically plausible, since all the output neurons display roughly similar variation in their firing, but Sanger's rule results in neurons whose behaviour is easier to interpret, since each neuron is tuned to a different component of the average stimulus. So, although a real nervous mechanism may work along the lines of an Oja network, it will be easier to understand if it is modelled by a Sanger network.

In practice, one cannot be sure of the average input correlation matrix of an actual neural mechanism, but one can sometimes determine the weighting functions of the output neurons. Such neural mechanisms have definitely not been trained by either the Oja rule or the Sanger rule, because they do not have orthogonal output weighting functions. However, by analogy with the formal neural networks a first step in understanding these weighting functions is to form the correlation matrix of the functions and then to compute the eigenvectors of the matrix. This method deriving a set of decorrelated weighting functions is referred to as the EIGENVECTOR TRANSFORMATION, and it will be used to understand both the colour and spatial coding mechanisms.

Summary

A linear filter has a set of inputs and one output. A weighting function specifies the relative strengths of each of the inputs. In the discrete case, there are n inputs $x_1, x_2, ...x_n$, with associated weights $w_1, w_2 ...w_n$, and the output y is given by the function:

$$y = \sum_{j=1}^{n} w_j x_j$$

The correlation matrix C is formed by the average of the correlations between each of the inputs..

Oja (1982) introduced a learning rule which ensures that the weights of the filter converge to the eigenvector of the input correlation matrix which has the largest eigenvalue. Let η be the learning rate factor, then the weight changes during training are specified by the equation:

$$\Delta w_j = \eta y (x_j - y w_j)$$

Sanger (1989) extended Oja's rule to networks containing more than one output. If the m outputs are indexed by the variable i then Sanger's rule can be written as:

$$\Delta w_{ij} = \eta y_i \left(x_j - \sum_{k=1}^{i} y_k w_{kj} \right)$$

In the networks produced by this rule, the weight vectors of successive outputs are equal to successive unit eigenvectors of the input correlation matrix.

By analogy with formal neural networks, real neural mechanisms can be understood by carrying out an eigenvector transformation, which involves forming the correlation matrix of the neural weighting functions and then computing the eigenvectors of the matrix. The eigenvectors specify a set of orthogonal weighting functions.

CHAPTER 8

Colour Coding

Colour vision provides a good starting point for investigating neural coding, because of the close agreement between psychophysical and neurophysiological findings. If an approach to understanding neural coding is to be viable, it must be successful with colour coding.

The Trichromatic Law

Many light sources can appear to have the same colour, despite having different wavelength distributions. This phenomenon can be investigated by COLOUR MATCHING. In a typical colour matching experiment the subject views a small stimulus which is usually restricted to around 2 degrees in diameter so that only the fovea is stimulated. The field is split into two halves and a pair of lights A and B, presented in one half, have to be matched in colour to a pair of lights C and D, presented in the other half. The main finding of colour matching experiments, referred to as the TRICHROMATIC LAW of colour matching, is that the colour of any stimulus can be matched by an additive mixture of three fixed primary colours.

The experimental findings can be described mathematically, by treating each colour stimulus as a vector, with the direction of the vector representing the qualitative nature of the colour and the size of the vector representing the amount of the colour. The base vectors $\mathbf{r}$, $\mathbf{g}$ and $\mathbf{b}$ are given by the functions of wavelengths $r(\lambda)$, $g(\lambda)$ and $b(\lambda)$ respectively, which describe the spectral power distribution of the fixed primary light sources. In vector notation, the trichromatic law states that any colour **c** can be matched by a linear combination of **r**, **g** and **b**:

$$c = r \ \mathbf{r} + g \ \mathbf{g} + b \ \mathbf{b}$$

If one of the coordinates r, g or b is negative, then one can move the term involved to the other side of the equation, to obtain a description of the physical situation where one pair of colours is matched by another pair.

In 1931, a standard colorimetric observer was defined by the 'Commission Internationale de l'Eclairage' (abbreviated to C.I.E.). The experimental results from many colour matching experiments were combined by expressing them all in terms of colour matches with three monochromatic light sources **r**, **g** and **b**, located at wavelengths of 700, 546.1 and 435.8 nm respectively. These wavelengths were chosen for ease of calibration of the physical light sources. The unit lengths of the vectors describing the light sources were set so that white was made by equal amounts of **r**, **g** and **b**. The coordinates $r\,(\lambda)$, $g\,(\lambda)$ and $b\,(\lambda)$ required to match a light with unit radiant power at wavelength λ, are a function of λ referred to as the COLOUR MATCHING FUNCTIONS. The colour matching functions which form the specification of the C.I.E. observer are plotted in Fig. 8.1.

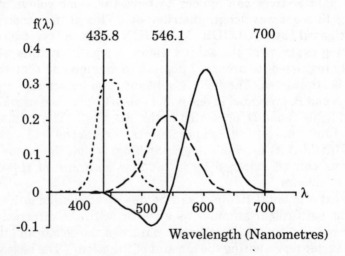

FIG. 8.1. Plot of $r\,(\lambda)$ (continuous line), $g\,(\lambda)$ (dashed line) and $b\,(\lambda)$ (dotted line) colour matching functions. The wavelengths of the r, g and b primary lights marked by vertical lines.

XYZ Colour Space

The direction of a colour vector can be isolated from its length by forming the intersection of the vector with a plane which passes through the 3 points specifying the unit distance along each base vector. For any set of (r, g, b) coordinates, one obtains a set of CHROMATICITY COORDINATES (r, g, b) such that r + g + b =1. The chromaticity coordinates are given by the formulae:

$$r r = \frac{r}{r +g +b}\, \mathbf{r}$$

$$g g = \frac{g}{r +g +b}\, \mathbf{g}$$

and

$$b b = \frac{b}{r +g +b}\, \mathbf{b}$$

Chromaticity coordinates can be plotted on a planar diagram by substituting geometrical vectors for **r**, **g** and **b**:

$$\mathbf{r} = (1, 0)$$
$$\mathbf{g} = (0, 1)$$
$$\mathbf{b} = (0, 0)$$

With these vectors, the locus of the chromaticity coordinates of the colour matching functions can be plotted on a chromaticity diagram, as shown in Fig. 8.2.

When defining their standard observer, the C.I.E. took the opportunity to simplify the chromaticity diagram. Negative chromaticity coordinates were eliminated by expressing the colour matching functions in terms of hypothetical primary lights referred to as **x**, **y** and **z**. Further simplification was achieved by selecting the lights so that one matched the luminance of the colour, and the other two made no contribution to the luminance match. In the **rgb** chromaticity diagram the line along which colours have zero luminance joins the points X and Z, marked on Fig. 8.2. The point Y was then selected so that the triangle XYZ is the smallest one which completely encloses the locus of the r (λ), g (λ) and b (λ) colour matching functions. One can then specify an **xyz** colour space, where the lights **x**, **y** and **z** correspond to the points X, Y and Z in the **rgb** chromaticity diagram.

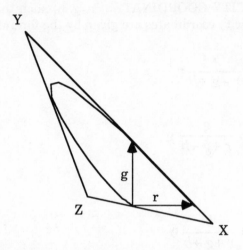

FIG. 8.2. Locus of the colour matching functions plotted on a chromaticity diagram. X, Y and Z mark the chromaticities of three hypothetical lights used in defining a simplified representation of the colour matching data.

The derivation of the XYZ colour space begins with three base vectors **x'**, **y'** and **z'** which have directions specified by the geometrical positions of the points X, Y and Z:

$$
\begin{bmatrix} \mathbf{x'} \\ \mathbf{y'} \\ \mathbf{z'} \end{bmatrix} = \begin{bmatrix} 1.275 & -0.278 & 0.003 \\ -1.74 & 2.768 & -0.028 \\ -0.743 & 0.141 & 1.602 \end{bmatrix} \begin{bmatrix} \mathbf{r} \\ \mathbf{g} \\ \mathbf{b} \end{bmatrix}
$$

inverting this matrix equation gives the **rgb** vectors in terms of the **x'y'z'** vectors:

$$\begin{bmatrix} r \\ g \\ b \end{bmatrix} = \begin{bmatrix} 0.909 & 0.091 & 0.0 \\ 0.575 & 0.419 & 0.006 \\ 0.371 & 0.005 & 0.624 \end{bmatrix} \begin{bmatrix} x' \\ y' \\ z' \end{bmatrix}$$

By definition, the colour white (denoted by **w**), is made by equal amounts of the **r**, **g** and **b** vectors, so one intensity of a white light is described by the equation:

$$w = 0.333r + 0.333g + 0.333b$$

Substituting for for **r**, **g** and **b** gives an equation for white in terms of **x'**, **y'** and **z'**:

$$w = 0.618x' + 0.1724y' + 0.21z'$$

In order to ensure that white is also made by equal amounts of **x**, **y** and **z**, one can put **x** = 0.539**x'**, **y** = 1.941**y'** and **z** = 1.587**z'**. It follows that the matrix equation which defines the **rgb** vectors in terms of the **xyz** vectors is:

$$\begin{bmatrix} r \\ g \\ b \end{bmatrix} = \begin{bmatrix} 0.49 & 0.177 & 0.0 \\ 0.31 & 0.812 & 0.01 \\ 0.2 & 0.011 & 0.99 \end{bmatrix} \begin{bmatrix} x \\ y \\ z \end{bmatrix}$$

As explained in chapter 3, if a matrix describes a change of basis, then the transpose of the matrix describes the change of coordinates, so that the relationship between coordinates in the two colour spaces is:

$$\begin{bmatrix} x \\ y \\ z \end{bmatrix} = \begin{bmatrix} 0.49 & 0.31 & 0.2 \\ 0.177 & 0.812 & 0.011 \\ 0.0 & 0.01 & 0.99 \end{bmatrix} \begin{bmatrix} r \\ g \\ b \end{bmatrix}$$

For convenience, the $y(\lambda)$ function, which describes how luminance varies with wavelength, is scaled to have a maximum of one. The x (λ), y (λ) and z (λ) colour matching functions are plotted in Fig. 8.3. and the corresponding chromaticity diagram is given in Fig. 8.4. Tabulated values of the colour matching functions can be found in Wright (1967), which also goes into the specification of the standard observer in greater detail.

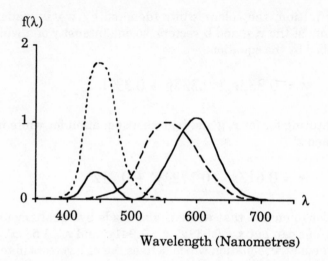

FIG. 8.3 The x (λ) (continuous line), y (λ) (dashed line) and z (λ) (dotted line) colour matching functions

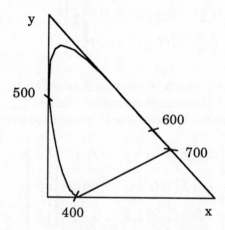

FIG. 8.4. The x (λ), y (λ) and z (λ) colour matching functions plotted in chromaticity space. The positions of spectral lights at 100 nanometre intervals are labelled.

Cone Sensitivities

The trichromatic law holds because there are only three types of cone, each of which responds best to a different wavelength. The results of colour matching experiments can be directly related to the properties of the cones, by expressing the results in a space spanned by the spectral sensitivity functions of the cones. This vector space is referred to as the **lms** space, corresponding to the three classes of cones with peaks in their spectral sensitivities at long, medium and short wavelengths respectively.

Vos and Walraven (1970) gave a comprehensive derivation of the **lms** space, a simplified version of which is given here. As with the transformation from the **rgb** to **xyz** sets of base vectors, the transformation from the **xyz** to the **lms** set of base vectors can be expressed as a matrix equation. One can determine the colour matching functions of the cones by setting up a matrix equation for the transformation of coordinates between the two colour spaces, which gives $x(\lambda)$, $y(\lambda)$ and $z(\lambda)$ in terms of $l(\lambda)$, $m(\lambda)$ and $s(\lambda)$:

$$\begin{bmatrix} x(\lambda) \\ y(\lambda) \\ z(\lambda) \end{bmatrix} = A \begin{bmatrix} l(\lambda) \\ m(\lambda) \\ s(\lambda) \end{bmatrix}$$

The normal observer, who requires three lights to match different colours, is referred to as TRICHROMATIC, and an observer who only requires two lights to match different colours is referred to as DICHROMATIC. The simplest assumption is that such an observer lacks one of the classes of cone and dichromats can be classified according to the class of cone which they lack.

PROTANOPES lack the long wavelength receptor. Since protanopes only require two lights for colour matching, values of x and y which are in a characteristic ratio will appear to have the same colour to the protanope and such values will lie along a line in the chromaticity diagram, referred to as a confusion line. Confusion lines formed by values in a fixed ratio all intersect at a point at which the output of both of the protanope receptors are zero. This point is referred to as the CONFUSION POINT. Some example confusion lines for protanopes, deuteranopes and tritanopes are shown in Figs. 8.5, 8.6 and 8.7 respectively.

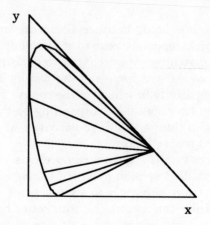

FIG. 8.5. Confusion lines of a protanope. The confusion point has chromaticity coordinates (0.747, 0.253, 0.0)

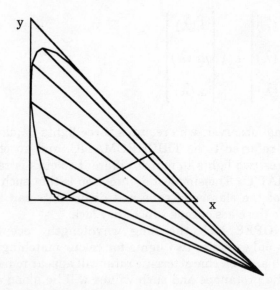

FIG. 8.6. Confusion lines of the deuteranope. The confusion point has chromaticity coordinates (1.4, -0.4, 0.0)

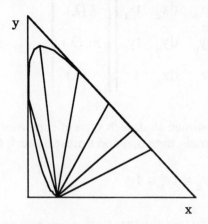

FIG. 8.7. Confusion lines of the tritanope. The confusion point has chromaticity coordinates (0.175, 0.004, 0.821)

At the protanopic confusion point, $m(\lambda) = s(\lambda) = 0$. If one could turn off these cone signals in a normal observer, then only the colour associated with the protanopic confusion point could be seen. This can only hold true if the first column of the matrix A is equal to a multiple of the chromaticity coordinates of the protanopic confusion point:

$$\begin{bmatrix} x \\ y \\ z \end{bmatrix} = \begin{bmatrix} px_p & a_{12} & a_{13} \\ py_p & a_{22} & a_{23} \\ pz_p & a_{32} & a_{33} \end{bmatrix} \begin{bmatrix} l(\lambda) \\ 0 \\ 0 \end{bmatrix}$$

where x_p, y_p and z_p are the coordinates of the protanopic confusion point and p is a scalar. Repeating this argument for the deuteranopic and tritanopic confusion points gives expressions for the remaining elements of the matrix A :

$$\begin{bmatrix} x\,(\lambda) \\ y\,(\lambda) \\ z\,(\lambda) \end{bmatrix} = \begin{bmatrix} px_p & dx_d & tx_t \\ py_p & dy_d & ty_t \\ pz_p & dz_d & tz_t \end{bmatrix} \begin{bmatrix} l\,(\lambda) \\ m\,(\lambda) \\ s\,(\lambda) \end{bmatrix}$$

If it is further assumed that each type of cone contributes directly to the luminance signal , then p, d and t must be such that:

$$py_p = dy_d = ty_t = 1$$

With these scale factors the transformation matrix becomes:

$$\begin{bmatrix} x\,(\lambda) \\ y\,(\lambda) \\ z\,(\lambda) \end{bmatrix} = \begin{bmatrix} 2.94 & -3.5 & 39.73 \\ 1.0 & 1.0 & 1.0 \\ 0.0 & 0.0 & 186.55 \end{bmatrix} \begin{bmatrix} l\,(\lambda) \\ m\,(\lambda) \\ s\,(\lambda) \end{bmatrix}$$

and the colour matching functions for this space can be obtained by inverting the matrix of the transformation:

$$\begin{bmatrix} l\,(\lambda) \\ m\,(\lambda) \\ s\,(\lambda) \end{bmatrix} = \begin{bmatrix} 0.1552 & 0.5431 & -0.036 \\ -0.1552 & 0.4569 & 0.0306 \\ 0.0 & 0.0 & 0.0054 \end{bmatrix} \begin{bmatrix} x\,(\lambda) \\ y\,(\lambda) \\ z\,(\lambda) \end{bmatrix}$$

The resulting spectral sensitivity curves of the cones are shown in Fig. 8.8. A logarithmic scale has been used because the s system of cones are so much less sensitive than the l and m systems of cones. The ratios of the maximum sensitivities of the l, m and s signals are 1: 0.5 : 0.025 respectively, and it is thought that these ratios reflect the relative number of the different types of cone in the retina. The scarcity of the s cones is supported by the findings of Bowmaker, Dartnall, Lythgoe and Mollon (1978) who measured the absorbance spectra of rods and cones in retinae taken from Rhesus monkeys.

When the absorption of the lens and the macula was taken into account, the curves were found to be similar to the psychophysical results. However, although they took measurements from 82 cones no s cones were found, only 42 m cones and 40 l cones.

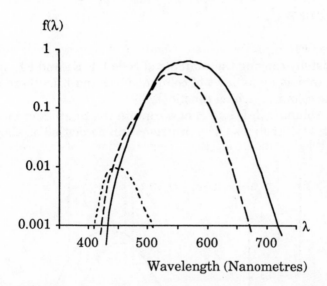

FIG. 8.8. Spectral sensitivities of the different cone types l (λ) (continuous line), m (λ) (dashed line) and s (λ) (dotted line)

Example Calculation: Smith and Pokorny Cone Sensitivity Functions

Smith and Pokorny (1975) derived an alternative set of cone sensitivity functions which are are often used in preference to the Vos and Walraven functions. Also, both groups actually defined their functions in terms of a standard observer which had been modified to correct for an underestimation of the sensitivity of the blue cones in the original C.I.E. observer.

Begin by entering the Judd modified values for the x (λ), y (λ) and $z(\lambda)$ colour matching functions into columns A,B and C of an Excel spreadsheet. A table of these values is given in Wysecki and Stiles (1975).

Next type in the following formulae:

= 0.15514*A1 + 0.54312*B1 - 0.03286*C1

into cell D1,

$$= -0.15514*A1 + 0.45684*B1 + 0.03286*C1$$

into cell E1, and

$$= 0.01608*C1$$

into cell F1.

Finish by copying the contents of cells D1, E1 and F1, and pasting them into as many rows of columns C, D and E as there are values for the colour matching functions.

The columns C, D and E now contain the Smith and Pokorny cone sensitivity functions. The functions can be plotted as shown in Fig. 8.9.

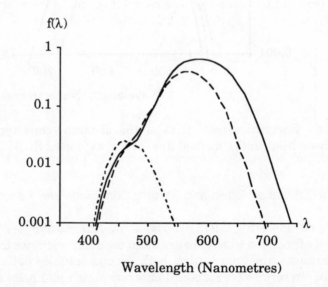

FIG. 8.9 Smith and Pokorny (1975) spectral sensitivity functions. The different classes of cones are plotted with the same types of line as in Fig. 8.8.

Opponent Colour Coding

The eigenvector transformation approach to understanding the implications of the cone sensitivity functions was introduced by Buchsbaum and Gottschalk (1983). For the cone sensitivity functions of Vos and Walraven, the correlation matrix of the sensitivity functions is:

$$\begin{bmatrix} c_{ll} & c_{lm} & c_{ls} \\ c_{ml} & c_{mm} & c_{ms} \\ c_{sl} & c_{sm} & c_{ss} \end{bmatrix} = \begin{bmatrix} 6.7231 & 3.3560 & 0.0038 \\ 3.3560 & 1.9887 & 0.0045 \\ 0.0038 & 0.0045 & 0.0008 \end{bmatrix}$$

If the three eigenvectors of the correlation matrix are written as rows of a matrix then a 3 x 3 matrix is obtained:

$$\begin{bmatrix} 0.8878 & 0.4602 & 0.0006 \\ 0.4602 & -0.8878 & -0.0090 \\ 0.0036 & -0.0083 & 0.9999 \end{bmatrix}$$

Multiplying the values of the cone sensitivity functions by the matrix of eigenvectors gives a set of decorrelated sensitivity functions, and these are plotted in Fig. 8.10.

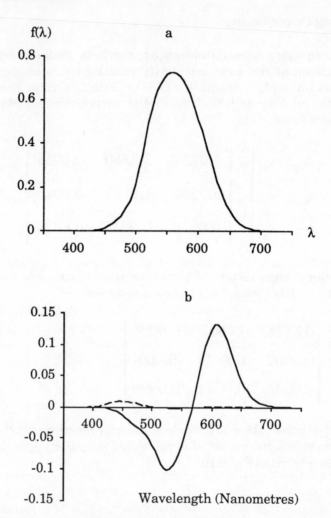

FIG. 8.10 Decorrelated spectral sensitivity functions produced by applying the eigenvector transformation to the cone sensitivity functions. a) Achromatic filter b) Chromatic filters. Red - Green (Continuous line) and Blue - Yellow (Broken line)

The upper trace in Fig. 8.10 corresponds to an achromatic luminance filter and so is referred to as the white - black filter. The middle trace corresponds to a red - green filter and the lower trace to a blue - yellow filter. The percentage of the variance of the cone signals which is carried by each filter is proportional to the eigenvalue associated with the eigenvector which defines the filter.

For the cone sensitivity functions the eigenvectors are:

[8.4628, 0.2491, 0.0008]

Clearly, the white - black filter carries most of the variance of the cone signals, the red - green filter carries the next largest proportion of the variance and the blue - yellow filter carries only a small proportion of the variance.

The eigenvector transformation reveals an opponent colour coding scheme which is in accord with subjective descriptions of colour appearance. One may see a greenish blue, but never a yellowish blue, and similarly one may see a yellowish green, but never a reddish green.

Example Calculation: The eigenvectors of the cone sensitivity functions correlation matrix.

Following on from the previous example, the correlations between each of the Smith and Pokorny (1975) cone spectral sensitivity functions can be calculated in the Excel spreadsheet. The correlation between the l and m cone functions can be calculated by typing:

= D1*E1

into cell G1, copying the entry and then pasting it into the remaining rows of column G, for which there are values in columns D and E. The correlation is obtained by summing all the values of all the cells in column G which are not empty. In this case the sum is equal to 1.6829.

The eigenvectors of the correlation matrix can be calculated using Mathematica. Begin by entering the elements of the correlation matrix c as a list of lists:

c = {{3.3623, 1.6829, 0.0069},
     {1.6829, 0.9951, 0.0069},
     {0.0069, 0.0069, 0.0031}}

Then simply type in:

Eigenvectors[c]

to obtain a list of the eigenvectors:

{{0.887487, 0.460827, 0.00219779},
{0.460734, -0.887189, -0.0248877},
{0.00951907, -0.0231001, 0.999688}}

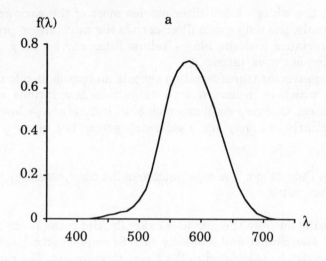

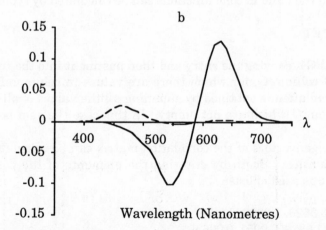

Wavelength (Nanometres)

FIG. 8.11. Decorrelated spectral sensitivity functions produced by applying the eigenvector transformation to the Smith and Pokorny (1975) cone sensitivity functions. As in Fig. 8.10, a) Achromatic filter b) Chromatic filters.

The linear combinations of the Smith and Pokorny sensitivity functions specified by these eigenvectors are plotted in Fig. 8.11 for comparison with the Vos and Walraven combinations plotted in Fig. 8.10.

Summary

Any colour can be matched by an additive mixture of three primary colours. Given three primary lights **x**, **y** and **z**, then the proportions of each light which are needed to match a unit radiant power light at wavelength l, are described by the colour matching functions $x(\lambda)$, $y(\lambda)$ and $z(\lambda)$.

If it assumed that colour anomalous observers lack one type of cone, then the confusion points of such observers can be used to determine the sensitivities of the different cone signals. The sensitivities of the l, m and s cones can be expressed in terms of the $x(\lambda)$, $y(\lambda)$ and $z(\lambda)$ colour matching functions by the transformation:

$$\begin{bmatrix} l(\lambda) \\ m(\lambda) \\ s(\lambda) \end{bmatrix} = \begin{bmatrix} 0.1552 & 0.5431 & -0.036 \\ -0.1552 & 0.4569 & 0.0306 \\ 0.0 & 0.0 & 0.0054 \end{bmatrix} \begin{bmatrix} x(\lambda) \\ y(\lambda) \\ z(\lambda) \end{bmatrix}$$

Application of the eigenvector transformation to the cone sensitivity functions produces a white - black filter, a red - green filter and a blue - yellow filter. The weighting functions of the filters are given by the matrix equation:

$$\begin{bmatrix} (w-b)(\lambda) \\ (r-g)(\lambda) \\ (b-y)(\lambda) \end{bmatrix} = \begin{bmatrix} 0.8878 & 0.4602 & 0.0006 \\ 0.4602 & -0.8878 & -0.009 \\ 0.0036 & -0.0083 & 0.9999 \end{bmatrix} \begin{bmatrix} l(\lambda) \\ m(\lambda) \\ s(\lambda) \end{bmatrix}$$

CHAPTER 9

Spatial Coding

It may seem perverse to begin a chapter on spatial coding with an outline of Fourier analysis, but the reason is simple. If one describes stimuli in terms of the spatial profile of their luminance, then it is not clear how one can relate the coding of one profile to that of another. Fourier analysis allows one to describe any function in terms of sinusoidal functions, so one can describe the differences between functions in terms of their respective Fourier components. This approach to spatial vision was pioneered by Campbell and Robson (1968).

Fourier Analysis

One way of producing a sinusoidal waveform is by calculating the projection onto a base vector of a vector to a point which is moving round a circle. This idea is illustrated in Fig. 9.1a, which shows a unit circle centred at the origin of a Cartesian system of axes. If the angle that the vector from the origin to the point z on the circle makes with the horizontal axis is denoted by q, then one can plot the projection of the rotating vector onto the horizontal axis as a function of θ, as shown in Fig. 9.1b.

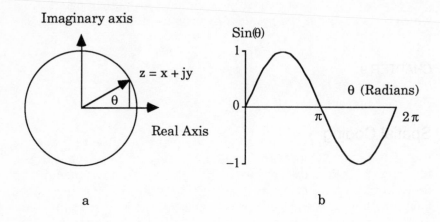

a   b

FIG. 9.1 Use of complex numbers in specifying a sinusoidal waveform. a) Specification of a point on a circle in the complex plane. b) Sinusoidal waveform corresponding to the projection of the point on the circle onto the real axis.

The position of the point on the circle which determines the generation of a sinusoidal waveform can be described by a complex number, which is a number consisting of the sum of a real part and an imaginary part. The use of the term imaginary is unfortunate, because it can be taken to mean that the number does not relate to actual events, whereas in fact complex numbers encapsulate the two dimensional nature of the mechanism underlying the generation of sinusoidal waveforms. The imaginary part of a complex number is a multiple of the imaginary number j which is defined to be equal to the square root of minus 1. Any complex number z can therefore be written in the form:

$$z = x + jy$$

where x is the real part and jy is the imaginary part. The two parts can be taken to specify a pair of plane Cartesian coordinates. By convention the real part is taken to represent the distance along the horizontal axis and the imaginary part is taken to represent the distance along the vertical axis, as shown in Fig. 9.1a.

The definition of the sine, cosine and exponential functions can be extended to complex versions of these functions by using power series representations of the functions. The defining property of the exponential function is that differentiation does not change it, from which it follows that the power series representation of the function is:

$$e^x = 1 + \frac{x}{1!} + \frac{x^2}{2!} + \frac{x^3}{3!} + \ldots$$

as differentiation of a term in the series gives the term to the left of the one being differentiated, so the series remains unchanged. Similarly, differentiation of the sine function gives the cosine function and differentiation of the cosine function gives the negative of the sine function, so the power series representations of these functions are:

$$\sin x = x - \frac{x^3}{3!} + \frac{x^5}{5!} - \ldots$$

and

$$\cos x = 1 - \frac{x^2}{2!} + \frac{x^4}{4!} - \ldots$$

The complex forms of these functions are defined by replacing the variable x with a complex variable z. The result of this substitution is that if one puts $z = 0 + jy$ then:

$$e^{jy} = 1 + \frac{jz}{1!} - \frac{z^2}{2!} - \frac{jz^3}{3!} + \frac{z^4}{4!} + \frac{jz^5}{5!} - \ldots$$

$$= (1 - \frac{z^2}{2!} + \frac{z^4}{4!} - \ldots) + j(z - \frac{z^3}{3!} + \frac{z^5}{5!} - \ldots)$$

$$= \cos y + j\sin y$$

so the plot of the function e^{jy} corresponds to the unit circle in the complex plane.

The Fourier representation of a function g(x) is obtained by combining the contributions of sinusoidal functions of all frequencies. Using the complex exponential functions to describe the sinusoidal functions gives an integral expression for the Fourier representation:

$$g(x) = \int_{-\infty}^{\infty} G(f) e^{j2\pi fx} df$$

where G(f) is the FOURIER TRANSFORM of the function g(x). The Fourier transform is evaluated according to the equation:

$$G(f) = \int_{-\infty}^{\infty} g(x) e^{-j2\pi fx} dx$$

If the expression for the Fourier transform is substituted for G(f) in the equation specifying the Fourier representation of g(x), then the exponential functions cancel out and g(x) is obtained, as required. Hence, the Fourier representation of g(x) is referred to as the INVERSE FOURIER TRANSFORM.

The function which arises most frequently in the context of neuronal operations is the Gaussian function:

$$g(x) = \frac{1}{\sigma\sqrt{2\pi}} e^{-\frac{1}{2}(\frac{x}{\sigma})^2}$$

where the parameter σ specifies how spread out the function is. The graph of a Gaussian with σ equal to one is plotted in Fig. 9.2.

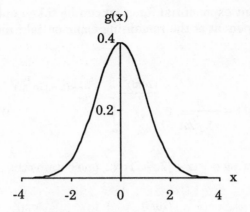

FIG. 9.2. Graph of a Gaussian function with $\sigma = 1$

The Gaussian function has the distinctive property that its Fourier transform is also a Gaussian function, as can be proved by evaluation of the transform. Substituting the Gaussian function in the definition of the transform gives the equation:

$$G(f) = \frac{1}{\sigma\sqrt{2\pi}} \int_{-\infty}^{\infty} e^{-\frac{1}{2}(\frac{x}{\sigma})^2} e^{-j2\pi fx} dx$$

The first stage in evaluating this integral involves combining the exponential functions:

$$G(f) = \frac{1}{\sigma\sqrt{2\pi}} \int_{-\infty}^{\infty} e^{-\frac{1}{2\sigma^2}(x^2 + j4\sigma^2\pi fx)} dx$$

The trick used to simplify the integral is to multiply and divide the exponential function by a quantity that enables one to factor the exponent of the function:

$$G(f) = \frac{1}{\sigma\sqrt{2\pi}} \int_{-\infty}^{\infty} e^{-\frac{(2\sigma\pi f)^2}{2}} e^{-\frac{1}{2\sigma^2}(x^2 + j4\sigma^2\pi fx - (2\sigma^2\pi f)^2)} dx$$

The constant exponential function can be taken outside the integral and the exponent of the remaining exponential function can then be factored:

$$G(f) = \frac{1}{\sigma\sqrt{2\pi}}\, e^{-\frac{(2\sigma\pi f)^2}{2}} \int_{-\infty}^{\infty} e^{-\frac{1}{2\sigma^2}(x + j2\sigma^2\pi f)^2}\, dx$$

Finally, putting $\sigma = (x + j2\sigma^2\pi f)/\sigma\sqrt{2}$, one obtains the result:

$$G(f) = \frac{1}{\sqrt{\pi}}\, e^{-\frac{(2\sigma\pi f)^2}{2}} \int_{-\infty}^{\infty} e^{-s^2}\, ds = e^{-\frac{(2\sigma\pi f)^2}{2}}$$

The final simplification relies on the knowledge that the value of the integral is $\sqrt{\pi}$. Simple numerical integration confirms this value. A graph of the real part of the Fourier transform of the Gaussian function plotted in Fig. 9.2 is shown in Fig. 9.3. The imaginary part of the transform is zero for every frequency.

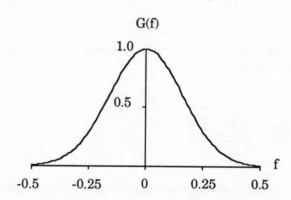

FIG. 9.3. Fourier transform of the Gaussian function plotted in Fig. 9.2.

Single Cell Neurophysiology

The RECEPTIVE FIELD of a single cell is defined to be the area of
the retina which must receive illumination to cause a discharge of
the cell. In the retina and lateral geniculate nucleus the receptive
fields of the cells have a concentric organisation consisting of a centre
and a surrounding ring. The centre responds to a stimulus being
turned either on or off, while the surrounding ring responds to a light
action that is opposite to that of the centre. The two areas of the
receptive field are mutually antagonistic, for if a light spot covers
both the centre and surround then the frequency of impulses is less
than for the centre or surround alone. The feature of the receptive
fields of cortical cells that distinguishes them from the receptive fields
of cells in the retina and lateral geniculate nucleus is that they are
elongated in one direction and so respond best to slits of light, dark
bars and edges. A distinction can be made between simple cells,
whose receptive fields can be explored with stationary spots of
flashing light, and complex cells which responded poorly to
stationary spots of flashing light. The receptive fields of simple cells
can be divided up into mutually exclusive regions, each of which
responds to light on or light off. Complex cells do not in general have
subdivisions of their receptive fields although they too are tuned to
stimuli with specific widths and orientations. Details of the
neurophysiology of the visual pathway can be found in Hubel (1988)

Enroth - Cugell and Robson (1966) investigated the assumption of
linear combination of inputs in visual neurons by recording the
responses of retinal ganglion cells to the presentation of stationary
gratings, and found that the behaviour of some of the cells
corresponded to that of a linear filter. Their procedure involved
moving the origin of the sinusoidal function defining the grating
across the receptive field of the cell in order to find a null position at
which there was no response. The existence of a null position implies
that linear combination of the inputs is occurring, as the input due to
the increase of light on one side of the origin is equal and opposite to
that due to the decrease of light on the other side of the origin. They
found that some retinal cells have a null position, whilst other cells do
not. This distinction between cells which show linear and cells which
show nonlinear spatial interaction also holds at the cortex; simple
cells are predominantly linear whilst complex cells are nonlinear.

Enroth - Cugell and Robson also found that the weighting function
of the linear neurons could be described by the difference between
two Gaussian functions of position. As shown in figure 9.4, the idea
behind their model is that both the centre and surround weightings

can be described by Gaussian functions. When the weighting of the inhibitory surround is summed with the centre weighting, the characteristic difference - of - Gaussian sensitivity profile is obtained.

Let s be the ratio of the σ of the centre to that of the surround, and let a and b scale the maximum values of the centre and surround respectively, then the weighting function w(x) of the receptive field in one dimension of a linear cell can be described by the equation:

$$w(x) = \frac{a}{\sigma\sqrt{2\pi}} e^{-\frac{1}{2}(\frac{x}{\sigma})^2} - \frac{b}{s\sigma\sqrt{2\pi}} e^{-\frac{1}{2}(\frac{x}{s\sigma})^2}$$

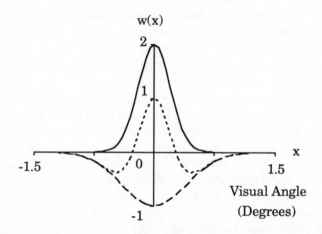

FIG. 9.4. Relative contributions of the centre and the surround to the difference - of - Gaussian model. The continuous line represents the weighting function of the centre, the dashed line represents the weighting function of the surround, and the dotted line specifies the resultant difference - of - Gaussian weighting function (a = b = 1, σ = 0.2, and s = 2).

One implication of the difference - of - Gaussian model is that the receptive fields will be tuned to a specific spatial freqency. On either side of the optimal spatial frequency, the response of the cell will drop off. The peak of the spatial frequency tuning curve of a cell with a receptive field profile described by this difference - of - Gaussian function can be calculated from the Fourier transform of the function. Application of the transform of a Gaussian derived in the previous section gives the Fourier transform of a difference - of -

Gaussian:

$$W(f) = ae^{-\frac{(2\sigma\pi f)^2}{2}} - be^{-\frac{(2s\sigma\pi f)^2}{2}}$$

Differentiating with respect to f, and using the constraint that at the optimal frequency W(f) = 0, gives the equation:

$$a(2\sigma\pi)^2 f \, e^{-\frac{(2\sigma\pi f)^2}{2}} = b(2s\sigma\pi)^2 f \, e^{-\frac{(2s\sigma\pi f)^2}{2}}$$

Taking the natural logarithm of both sides of the equation:

$$\ln(a) + \ln((2\sigma\pi)^2 f) - \frac{(2\sigma\pi f)^2}{2} =$$

$$\ln(bs^2) + \ln((2\sigma\pi)^2 f) - \frac{(2s\sigma\pi f)^2}{2}$$

Collecting like terms gives the simpler equation:

$$\frac{(2\sigma\pi f)^2 (s^2 - 1)}{2} = \ln(bs^2) - \ln(a)$$

From which it follows that the peak frequency is given by the quadratic equation:

$$f = \sqrt{\frac{\ln(\frac{bs^2}{a})}{(\sqrt{2}\,\sigma\pi)^2 (s^2 - 1)}}$$

This formula gives a peak frequency of 0.765 cycles per degree for the difference - of - Gaussian function plotted in Fig. 9.4. The complete transform is plotted in Fig. 9.5.

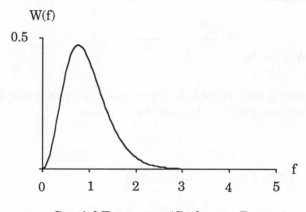

Spatial Frequency (Cycles per Degree)

FIG. 9.5. Fourier transform of the difference - of - Gaussian function plotted in Fig. 9.4. The peak frequency is at 0.765 cycles per degree.

Curves with similar shapes can be obtained from real cells by averaging their responses to gratings drifting across their receptive fields. Typically, the centre is stronger than the surround so that the cell responds even to very low frequencies.

As well as describing the properties of simple and complex cells, Hubel and Wiesel (1962) also proposed a simple wiring diagram to explain the properties of the cells. According to their scheme retinal cells connect to cells in the lateral geniculate nucleus, and the on regions of simple cells are formed by connecting up rows of on centre cells in the lateral geniculate nucleus, and similarly the off regions are formed by connecting up rows of off centre cells in the lateral geniculate nucleus. For cells which show linear spatial summation over their receptive fields, this scheme agrees with the experimental findings, so the natural extension of the difference - of - Gaussian to simple cells involves modelling each separate on and off region by a difference - of - Gaussian function. Hawken and Parker (1987) tested this extension of the model by measuring the spatial frequency tuning curves of cortical cells in the monkey, and fitting the curves with the Fourier transform of a receptive field model made up of spatially separated difference - of - Gaussian functions. Their results made it clear that many simple cells have asymmetric receptive fields, in which an on region on one side is much stronger than the corresponding region on the other side. In order to understand what use is made of the output from such cells with asymmetric receptive fields, their combined outputs have to be investigated psychophysically.

Example Calculation: Quadrature filters

Typically, the frequency tuning of a neuron is determined by measuring the response of the neuron to a drifting sinusoidal grating over a range of frequencies. However, this tuning curve does not provide enough information to specify the spatial weighting function of the neuron because it does not tell one how the response of the neuron depends on the position of the grating within its receptive field.

If the generation of a sinusoidal function is thought of in terms of the projection of a point moving around a circle, as was portrayed in Fig. 9.1, then the AMPLITUDE of the sinusoidal function corresponds to the radius of the circle and the PHASE of the sinusoidal function corresponds to the angle between the line to the point and the horizontal axis. When the position of the point is described by a complex number z = x + jy, then the amplitude and phase associated with the position are:

$$\text{Amplitude} = \sqrt{x^2 + y^2}$$

and

$$\text{Phase} = \text{Arctan}(\frac{y}{x})$$

The difference - of - Gaussian function is symmetric about the origin, and hence all of its sinusoidal components consist of cosine waves, which are also symmetric about the origin. Clearly, a function could be made up entirely of sine waves, each with an amplitude equal to that of the cosine wave with the same frequency. This function would be anti - symmetric in that for any x it would hold that f(x) = - f(x), since the function is composed entirely of sine waves which are themselves anti - symmetric. Any pair of functions which have the same amplitude against frequency profile, but which have phases that are ninety degrees apart are referrred to as QUADRATURE PAIRS. An example of a quadature pair of filters is shown in Fig. 9.6. The symmetric function is a difference - of -

Gaussian with a centre σ of 0.04 and a surround σ of 0.08. The associated anti - symmetric function was calculated using the most recent version of Excel, which includes a Fourier transform routine.

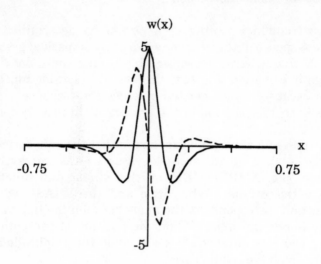

Figure 9.6. Weighting functions of a pair of quadrature filters

The first thing to realise, before beginning the calculation, is that the number of data points must be a power of two for the Fourier routine to work. This is because numerical Fourier transforms involve successively splitting up the data. The second point is that the numerical Fourier transform does not go from minus an infinitely large frequency to plus an infinitely large frequency, as required by the analytical definition of a Fourier transform.. Rather the positive frequency components come first and the negative frequency components form the second half of the transform. The difference between the two transforms is simplest to understand graphically. A 64 point numerical Fourier transform of the difference - of - Gaussian function is shown in Fig. 9.7. The first step in producing this transform is to type in whole numbers in the range 0 through to 31 in successive rows of the first column of the spreadsheet, followed by whole numbers in the range 32 through to 1 in the following rows. In effect, the 64 numbers in this column specify the frequency range to be from 0 to 32 cycles. The analytical formula for the transform of the difference - of Gaussian is then pasted into the first 64 cells of the next column. In the first cell (B1) the function reads:

```
=EXP(-0.5*(2*0.04*PI()*A1)^2)
    -EXP(-0.5*(2*0.08*PI()*A1)^2)
```

It is the contents of this column which are plotted in Fig. 9.7.

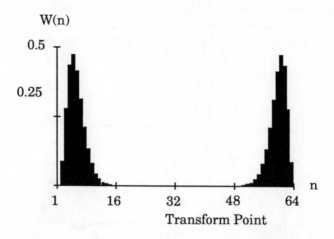

Figure 9.7. Numerical Fourier transform of the difference - of - Gaussian function plotted in Fig. 9.6.

The numerical Fourier transform of the associated anti - symmetric function is simply formed by putting the imaginary part of the transform to be equal to the real part of the transform of the symmetric function. The only complication is that because the second half of the transform corresponds to negative frequencies, the sign of these transform points must be reversed. In terms of the spreadsheet, all that is involved is to type :

```
= COMPLEX(0, B1)
```

into the first cell in column C and then to copy and paste this entry into the next 31 cells. Type:

```
= COMPLEX(0, -B1)
```

into cell C33 and then copy and paste this entry into all the cells up to C64. (I found that to make the Fourier analysis routine work, at this point I had to go back and change the entry in cell C1 to:

```
=COMPLEX(0,B1+0.00000000000001)
```

The change does not significantly affect the outcome of the computation)

The rest is easy. Select the first 64 cells in column C, choose Analysis Tools from the options menu, and then go on to to choose Fourier Analysis from the list of Analysis Tools. Type in D1 to place the results in column D and click in the inverse transform box. The numerical inverse transform of the anti - symmetric filter appears as shown in Fig. 9.8. The anti - symmetric function plotted in figure 9.6 was obtained by putting the data points of the numerical inverse transform into the right order.

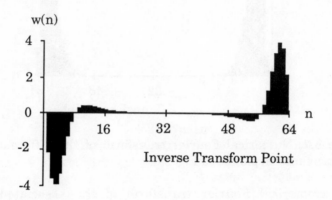

Figure 9.8. Inverse numerical Fourier transform of the anti - symmetric filter.

Spatial Frequency Selectivity

Blakemore and Campbell (1969) found that spatially tuned mechanisms in the human visual system could be revealed by studying the aftereffects of prolonged viewing of a high contrast sinusoidal grating. The subject viewed a high contrast grating at a fixed frequency for one minute, prior to viewing a low contrast test grating. The task of the observer was to adjust the contrast of the test grating until it was just visible. Using this technique the elevation of the threshold sensitivity curve around the adapting frequency could be measured. The threshold elevation curve has its peak at the adapting frequency, and falls off on either side of the adapting frequency. This finding suggests that the spatially tuned mechanism underlying the effect acts as a filter which only lets a range of frequencies past.

A measure of the range of frequencies which a filter will pass is given by its half - height, half - width parameter. This is determined by the difference between the peak frequency of the filter and the frequency at which the response of the filter to unit amplitude sinusoidal gratings has dropped to one half of its maximum. On a logarithmic scale the separation between a given frequency and half the given frequency is the same as the distance between the given frequency and double the given frequency, and this separation of frequencies is referred to as an OCTAVE. A characteristic of the threshold elevation curves is that they all have approximately the same symmetrical shape when plotted on a logarithmic scale, with a half - height, half - width of one octave. These characteristic Fourier representations can be modelled by the Fourier transform of a difference - of - Gaussian function in which the s of the surround is double that of the centre, and examples of the weighting functions of some of these filters are plotted in Fig 9.9. Interestingly, the adaptation aftereffect was found to be orientation sensitive, which implies that cortical neurons are involved.

Application of the eigenvector transformation to the spatial frequency filters involves many more than three filters, but as more filters are modelled the overlap becomes greater and the contribution of the additional filters becomes less. As an example, one can use the four filters shown in Fig 9.9 as a model of the spatial coding mechanism.

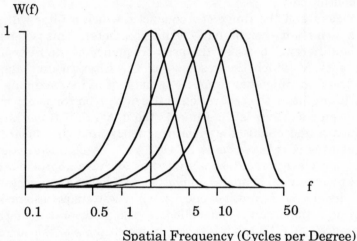

Spatial Frequency (Cycles per Degree)

FIG. 9.9. Difference - of - Gaussian models of the spatial frequency tuned filters found psychophysically. Filters tuned to frequencies of 2, 4, 8 and 16 cycles per degree are shown. The optimum frequency of the 2 cycle per degree filter is marked by a vertical line, and the octave half - height, half - width of the filter is marked with a horizontal line.

The correlation matrix C of the four filters is:

$$
C = \begin{bmatrix}
1.93 & 1.337 & 0.5087 & 0.1466 \\
1.337 & 1.93 & 1.3318 & 0.5121 \\
0.5087 & 1.3318 & 1.93 & 1.3426 \\
0.1466 & 0.5121 & 1.3426 & 1.93
\end{bmatrix}
$$

and the first three eigenvectors of this matrix account for 98% of the variance of the output of the correlated filters. The Fourier transforms of these eigenvectors are plotted in Fig. 9.10 and the corresponding weighting functions are plotted in Fig. 9.11.

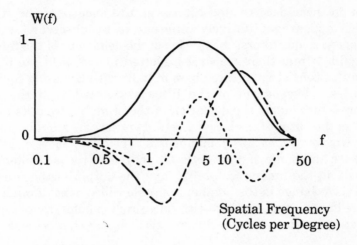

FIG. 9.10 Fourier transforms of the 3 largest decorrelated spatial frequency channels. In this and the following 2 figures, the continuous line corresponds to the largest eigenvector, the dashed line to the next largest eigenvector and the dotted line to the third largest eigenvector.

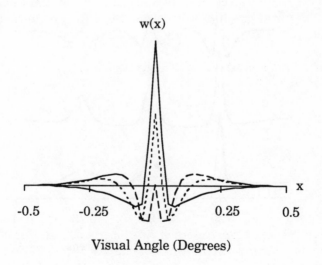

FIG. 9.11. Relative sizes of the weighting functions of the decorrelated spatially - tuned filters.

So do these decorrelated filters capture aspects of the stimulus which appear qualitatively different to an observer, as do the opponent colour filters? Some idea of the behaviour of the filters can be gained from their responses, plotted in Fig. 9.12., to a simple stimulus consisting of three bars of light with Gaussian luminance profiles. The output of the filter associated with the largest eigenvector signals the deviation of the stimulus from its average, and so the output falls below zero in between the stimulus bars. In terms of sensations, any point appears to be either above or below the average luminance, but not both. The output of the next filter signals a peak in the luminance profile, and the output of the third filter signals a change in the luminance profile which is not a minimum or a maximum. If the analogy with colour coding holds, these aspects of the stimulus constitute the dimensions along which it is coded.

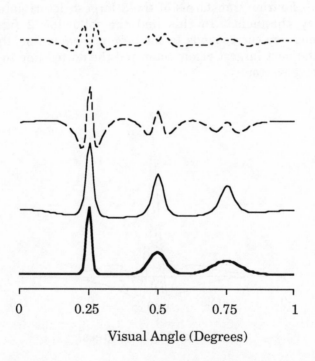

Visual Angle (Degrees)

FIG. 9.12 Relative responses of the decorrelated filters to a stimulus consisting of three light bars. For comparison, the luminance profile of the stimulus is plotted as a bold line at the bottom of the figure.

Spatiochromatic Coding

Although colour and spatial coding has been treated separately, visual cells make no such distinction. The receptive fields of simple colour opponent cells have an antagonistic centre - surround organisation when tested with small spots of white light. But when a large spot of monochromatic light is used, then it is found that at some point along the wavelength scale a cell ceases to be excited by the stimulus and instead is inhibited. An instructive model for the organisation of the receptive field of an l - m colour opponent cell, which is excited by red in its centre and inhibited by green in its surround, was developed by Ingling and Martinez - Uriegas (1983). If a difference - of - Gaussian with a 1:2 centre:surround ratio is used to model the weighting profile of the cell, then the receptive field and its associated weighting function appear as shown in Fig.9.13.

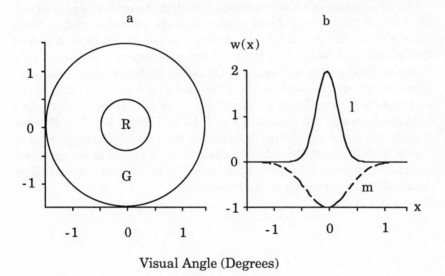

Visual Angle (Degrees)

FIG. 9.13. Receptive field of a colour opponent cell. a) Concentric organisation of receptive field. b) Cone weighting functions associated with a cross - section of the receptive field. The same labels are used in Fig. 9.14 and Fig. 9.15.

At any visual angle x with respect to the centre of the receptive field, the spectral sensitivity of the cell will be:

$$f(\lambda) = g_c(x)l\,(\lambda) - g_s(x)m\,(\lambda)$$

where $g_c(x)$ and $g_s(x)$ are the Gaussian functions which describe the weighting of the centre and surround respectively. Ingling and Martinez - Uriegas pointed out that this equation can be factorised:

$$f(\lambda) = \frac{(g_c(x) - g_s(x))}{2}\,(l\,(\lambda) + m\,(\lambda)) +$$

$$\frac{(g_c(x) + g_s(x))}{2}\,(l\,(\lambda) - m\,(\lambda))$$

The implication of this factorisation is that the colour opponent cell mechanism can be considered to consist of the sum of a white - black filter with a red - green filter, and that, the two filters have different spatial characteristics. The white - black component is mediated by a receptive field with a difference of Gaussian profile. whereas the red - green component is mediated by a receptive field with a profile given by the sum of two Gaussian functions. The two different receptive field mechanisms are shown in Fig. 9.14 and Fig. 9.15. The Fourier transforms of the weighting functions of the two channels, plotted in Fig. 9.16, show that the white - black filter is tuned to an optimum spatial frequency, whereas the sensitivity of the red - green filter drops off with increasing spatial frequency.

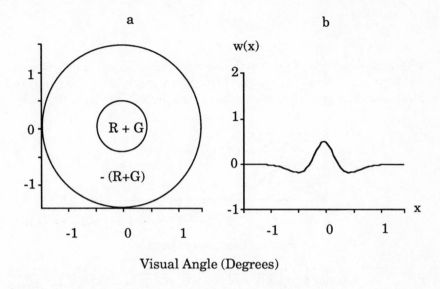

FIG. 9.14. White - black component of the receptive field of a colour opponent cell.

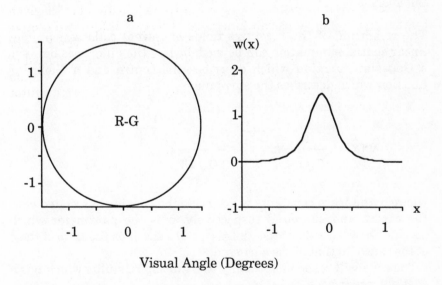

FIG. 9.15. Red - green component of the receptive field of a colour opponent cell.

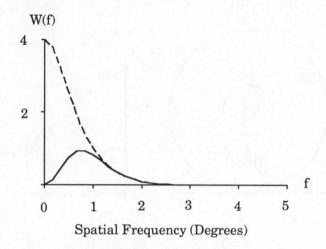

FIG. 9.16. Fourier transforms of the weighting functions of the white - black (continuous line) and red - green (broken line) mechanisms.

Summary

The weighting of the receptive fields of retinal cells which show linear spatial summation can be modelled by the difference between a Gaussian function which describes the centre and a Gaussian function which describes the surround:

$$w(x) = \frac{a}{\sigma\sqrt{2\pi}} e^{-\frac{1}{2}(\frac{x}{\sigma})^2} - \frac{b}{s\sigma\sqrt{2\pi}} e^{-\frac{1}{2}(\frac{x}{s\sigma})^2}$$

where a and b are constants which scale the weights associated with the centre and surround respectively, σ is the parameter which specifies how spread out the centre is, and s specifies the ratio of the σ of the centre to that of the surround.

The cells will respond optimally to a grating stimulus which has a spatial frequency of:

$$f = \sqrt{\frac{\ln(\frac{bs^2}{a})}{(\sqrt{2}\,\sigma\pi)^2(s^2 - 1)}}$$

The spatial frequency filters found psychophysically can be modelled by difference - of - Gaussian functions in which the ratio s of the surround σ to the centre σ is 2.   The eigenvector transformation results in decorrelated spatial frequency filters which encode the deviation of the luminance from its spatial average, peaks in the luminance profile, and changes in the luminance profile which are neither minima nor maxima.

CHAPTER 10

Mechanical Systems

As this book is concerned with the stimulus transformations that occur along the visual pathway, discussion of the motor image will be restricted to the commands involved in eye movement specification. In order to investigate the signals used to control eye movements one has to be able to calculate the rotation of the eye that follows a given input to the eye muscles This chapter introduces the linear system approach to the calculation of the responses of mechanical systems.

Equations of mechanical systems

The behaviour of simple mechanical systems can be described by a TRANSFER FUNCTION which specifies the output of the system in terms of its input. If x(t) is a function of time t which describes the input to the system and y(t) is a function, also of time, which describes the output of the system, then the transfer function H is given by the ratio:

$$H(t) = \frac{y(t)}{x(t)}$$

The simplest mechanical system is one in which the output y is directly proportional to the input x. If k is the constant of proportionality then the transfer function of this system is:

$$\frac{y(t)}{x(t)} = k$$

The next simplest mechanical system is one in which the output y and its rate of change are both proportional to the input x. Let k be as before and a_1 be the constant of proportionality describing the relationship between the first derivative of y and kx. The general equation of such a system is:

$$a_1\frac{dy(t)}{dt} + y(t) = kx(t)$$

The transfer function of this system is:

$$\frac{y(t)}{x(t)} = \frac{k}{(a_1\frac{d}{dt} + 1)}$$

The most complicated mechanical system that will be used here is one in which the output y, its rate of change and its rate of change of rate of change all depend on the input x. The equation for this system is:

$$a_2\frac{d^2y(t)}{dt} + a_1\frac{dy(t)}{dt} + y(t) = kx(t)$$

and the system has the transfer function:

$$\frac{y(t)}{x(t)} = \frac{k}{(a_2(\frac{d}{dt})^2 + a_1\frac{d}{dt} + 1)}$$

where a_2 is the constant of proportionality describing the relationship between the second derivative of y and kx. These systems are examples of zero, first and second order types respectively; the type of the system being determined by the highest power of the derivative in the transfer function.

The equations which describe the behaviour of such mechanical systems can be solved by the application of calculus, but it is simpler to transform the equations so that they can be solved by algebraic manipulation. The transformation is referred to as the LAPLACE TRANSFORM and involves evaluating the integral of the function to be transformed with a complex exponential. If the transform is denoted by L then:

$$L\,[f(t)] = \int_0^\infty f(t)e^{-st}dt$$

The transfer functions of the zero, first and second order systems given at the beginning of the section can be rewritten using Laplace transforms as:

$$\frac{Y(s)}{X(s)} = k$$

$$\frac{Y(s)}{X(s)} = \frac{k}{a_1s + 1}$$

and

$$\frac{Y(s)}{X(s)} = \frac{k}{a_2s^2 + a_1s + 1}$$

where $X(s)$ and $Y(s)$ are the Laplace transforms of the input and output functions respectively. The only second order systems which will be applied to the oculomotor mechanism are ones which can be considered as two first order systems in series, so that the transfer function can be factorised:

$$\frac{Y(s)}{X(s)} = \frac{k}{(b_1s + 1)(b_2s + 1)}$$

where $b_1b_2 = a_2$ and $b_1 + b_2 = a_1$.

In the next section the most commonly used Laplace transforms will be derived. The section is included primarily for completeness, the main import of the chapter being contained in the section in which the responses of the mechanical systems are derived.

Basic Laplace Transforms

For some of the simpler functions, calculation of the Laplace transform is straightforward. A useful function for determining the properties of such systems is the IMPULSE FUNCTION, which is an idealised function that approaches an infinite value and returns again to zero all in one instant. A description of the function is obtained by treating it as a limiting case of the rectangular function shown in Fig. 10.1. The rectangular function starts at time t = 0, immediately reaches a value 1/a, remains constant until t = a and then immediately returns to the zero value. The area under the graph of the function is unity and as a is brought closer to zero, the duration of the impulse function tends to zero, so the complex exponential function is equal to unity. Hence

$$\mathcal{L}\,[f(t)] = 1$$

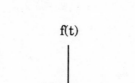

FIG. 10.1 The rectangular function

The STEP FUNCTION arises when a variable is zero and then at some instant takes a value c, but is constant after the change. This is shown in Fig. 10.2, where the change is taken to occur at time $t = 0$.

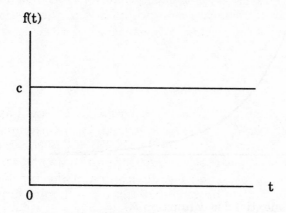

FIG. 10.2 The step function

$$\mathcal{L}\,[f(t)] = \int_0^\infty ce^{-st}dt = \left[\frac{ce^{-st}}{s}\right]_0^\infty = 0 - \left(\frac{c}{s}\right) = \frac{c}{s}$$

The EXPONENTIAL DECAY function is defined by the equation:

$$f(t) = \frac{c}{T}\,e^{-\frac{t}{T}}$$

and a graph of the function is given in Fig. 10.3.

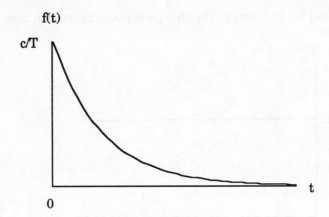

FIG. 10.3 The exponential decay function

$$L [f(t)] = \int_0^\infty \frac{c}{T} e^{-\frac{t}{T}} e^{-st} dt = \int_0^\infty \frac{c}{T} e^{-(\frac{1}{T} + s)t} dt$$

$$= \left[\frac{c}{Ts + 1} e^{-(\frac{1}{T} + s)t} \right]_0^\infty = \frac{c}{Ts + 1}$$

The counterpart to the decay function is the EXPONENTIAL GROWTH function which is described by the equation:

$$f(t) = \frac{c}{T} (1 - e^{-\frac{t}{T}})$$

The graph of this function is shown in Fig. 10.4.

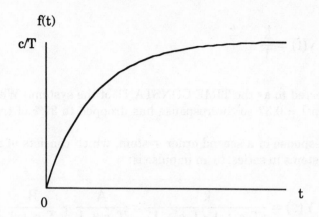

FIG. 10.4. The exponential growth function

$$\mathcal{L}\,[f(t)] = \int\limits_0^\infty \frac{c}{T}\,(1 - e^{-\frac{t}{T}})\,e^{-st}dt$$

$$= \int\limits_0^\infty \frac{c}{T}\,e^{-st}dt - \int\limits_0^\infty -\frac{c}{T}\,e^{-(\frac{1}{T} + s)t}\,dt$$

$$= \frac{c}{Ts} - \frac{c}{Ts + 1} = \frac{\dfrac{c}{T}}{s(Ts + 1)}$$

Responses of Mechanical Systems

The response of the first order system specified in the first section to an impulse is:

$$Y(s) = \frac{k}{Ts + 1}$$

which is the Laplace transform of a decaying exponential:

$$y(t) = \frac{k}{T} e^{-\frac{t}{T}}$$

T is referred to as the TIME CONSTANT of the system. When $t = T$ then $\exp^{-1} = 0.37$ so the response has dropped to 37% of the initial input.

The response of a second order system, which consists of two first order systems in series, to an impulse is:

$$Y(s) = \frac{k}{(T_1 s + 1)(T_2 s + 1)} = \frac{A}{T_1 s + 1} + \frac{B}{T_2 s + 1}$$

In order to evaluate A multiply both sides of the equation by the denominator of A:

$$\frac{k}{T_2 s + 1} = A + \frac{B(T_1 s + 1)}{T_2 s + 1}$$

and put $s = -1/T_1$ so that the term involving B disappears:

$$A = \frac{k}{1 - \dfrac{T_2}{T_1}}$$

Similarly, B can be evaluated by multiplying both sides of the equation by the denominator of B and putting $s = -1/T_2$ so that the term involving A disappears. The expression for B given by this procedure is:

$$B = \frac{k}{1 - \dfrac{T_1}{T_2}}$$

Hence the Laplace transform of the impulse function can be rewritten as:

$$Y(s) = \frac{k}{(T_1 s + 1)(1 - \frac{T_2}{T_1})} - \frac{k}{(T_2 s + 1)(1 - \frac{T_1}{T_2})}$$

which is the Laplace transform of the sum of two exponential functions:

$$y(t) = \frac{T_1}{(T_1 - T_2)} \frac{k}{T_1} e^{-\frac{t}{T_1}} + \frac{T_2}{(T_2 - T_1)} \frac{k}{T_2} e^{-\frac{t}{T_2}}$$

$$= \frac{k}{T_1 - T_2} (e^{-\frac{t}{T_1}} - e^{-\frac{t}{T_2}})$$

An example plot of this function is shown in Fig. 10.5. Effectively the output of the system is a smeared pulse.

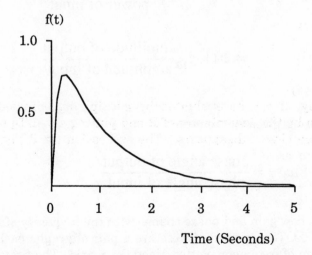

FIG. 10.5. Example of the impulse response of a second order system when $k = 1$, $T_1 = 1$ and $T_2 = 0.1$ seconds.

Bode Plots

To appreciate the behaviour of mechanical systems it is simplest to consider the way in which the systems respond to a sinusoidal input. Since differentiation of a sinusoidal waveform does not alter the frequency of the waveform, the first and second order systems can only alter the amplitude and phase of the sinusoidal signal, they cannot alter its frequency. Hence two functions can be used to describe the properties of the systems. The first is the GAIN, which relates the amplitude of the output to the amplitude of the input, and the second is PHASE, which relates the phase of the output to the phase of the input.

The basic unit of gain is the bel which is such that a tenfold increase in power corresponds to a gain of 1 bel. However, a more useful quantity is the DECIBEL (abbreviated to dB) which is a subdivision of the bel such that a tenfold increase in power corresponds to a gain of 10dB. The emphasis on power in the definition of a bel originates with its use by electrical engineers. In signal processing applications, it is usually the amplitude of the signal that is of interest. Since the power of a signal is given by the square of its amplitude, gain in dB can be defined directly in terms of the amplitudes of the input and output:

$$\text{gain (in db)} = 10 \log_{10} \frac{\text{power of output}}{\text{power of input}}$$

$$= 20 \log_{10} \frac{\text{amplitude of output}}{\text{amplitude of input}}$$

The phase is given by the ratio:

$$\text{Phase} = \frac{\text{phase angle of output}}{\text{phase angle of input}}$$

To show how gain and phase change with the frequency of the signal, BODE PLOTS are used. These are a pair of graphs each with the logarithm of frequency plotted along the x axis. The first graph has the gain in dB plotted along the y axis, whilst the second graph has the phase angle in degrees plotted along the y axis.

The response of a system as a function of frequency can be determined by putting s = (0 + jw) where w is the angular frequency $2\pi f$ so that e^{-st} corresponds to rotation of a point about the unit circle in the complex plane.

For a first order system:

$$\frac{Y(s)}{X(s)} = \frac{k}{Ts + 1}$$

becomes:

$$\frac{Y(j\omega)}{X(j\omega)} = \frac{k}{Tj\omega + 1}$$

The amplitude of a complex sinusoidal signal is given by the square root of the sum of the squares of the real and imaginary parts, so the gain is given by:

$$\left|\frac{Y(\omega)}{X(\omega)}\right| = 20 \log_{10} \left(\frac{k}{\sqrt{T^2\omega^2 + 1}}\right)$$

and the gain plot for a system with steady state gain of one (k = 1) and a time constant of unity (T = 1) is plotted in Fig. 10.6.

When the frequency of the sinusoidal input is low, then the contribution of the T^2w^2 term is negligible and the gain of the system equals 0. When the frequency is high, then only the contribution of the T^2w^2 term matters and the gain equals $-20\log_{10}T - 20\log_{10}w$. If a tenfold increase in frequency is referred to as a decade then it follows that the slope of the asymptote to the high frequency portion of the curve is -20dB per decade. If one is investigating a system whose transfer function is not known, then one can approximate the gain curve with straight line segments, each of which has a 20 dB increase in slope, and deduce from the number of breaks in the curve the order of the system.

The intersection of the asymptote of the curve (drawn on the figure with a dashed line) with the frequency axis occurs when the frequency f is such that $2\pi f = 1 / T$, which in this case is when f =1/ 2π = 0.16 hz. At this frequency, the amplitude of the output is half that of the input, and the gain has the value - 20 $\log_{10} \sqrt{1/2}$, which equals -3dB.

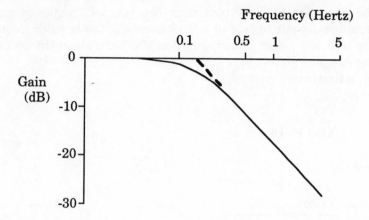

FIG. 10.6. Gain plot for a first order system with a time constant of one. An extension of the high frequency asymptote to the frequency axis is represented by a dashed line. The asymptote intersects the axis at a frequency of $1/2\pi T$.

The phase is given by the inverse tangent of the ratio of imaginary to real parts, so

$$\angle \frac{Y(j\omega)}{X(j\omega)} = -\arctan \omega T$$

The negative sign is chosen to indicate that the output is lagging behind the input. The phase plot of a first order system with a time constant of unity is shown in Fig. 10.7. The frequency $f = 1/2\pi T$ is also significant in the context of phase, in that it is associated with a 45 degree phase lag.

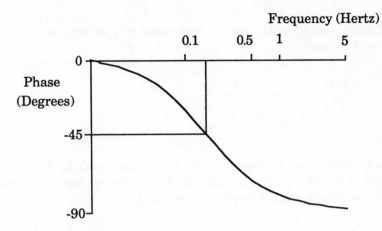

FIG. 10.7. Phase plot of a first order system

For two first order systems in sequence the gains combine multiplicatively:

$$\left|\frac{Y(\omega)}{X(\omega)}\right| = 20 \log_{10}\left(\frac{k}{\sqrt{T_1^2\omega^2 + 1}\sqrt{T_2^2\omega^2 + 1}}\right)$$

and the phases combine additively:

$$\angle\frac{Y(j\omega)}{X(j\omega)} = -\arctan \omega T_1 - \arctan \omega T_2$$

Summary

The transfer function of a system relates its output y(t) to its input x(t). For a simple first order system the transfer function is:

$$\frac{y(t)}{x(t)} = \frac{k}{T\dfrac{d}{dt} + 1}$$

and for a second order system comprised of two simple first order systems in series:

$$\frac{y(t)}{x(t)} = \frac{k}{(T_1\frac{d}{dt} + 1)(T_2\frac{d}{dt} + 1)}$$

The behaviour of a linear system is characterised by its impulse response function. For the simple first order system the impulse response function is a decaying exponential:

$$y(t) = \frac{k}{T} e^{-\frac{t}{T}}$$

The significance of the time constant T is that it is the time after which the impulse response drops to 37% of its initial value. The impulse response of two simple first order linear systems in series is given by the difference of two exponential decay functions:

$$y(t) = \frac{k}{T_1 - T_2} (e^{-\frac{t}{T_1}} - e^{-\frac{t}{T_2}})$$

CHAPTER 11

One - Dimensional Eye Movements

Phylogenically, the oldest oculomotor mechanism is the reflex which acts to hold the gaze steady despite movements of the head. Investigation of this reflex shows that there must exist a neural circuit which converts eye velocity to eye position, and this circuit is also involved in the control of voluntary changes in gaze direction.

Mechanics of the Semicircular Canals

Movements of the head are signalled by the semicircular canals. A diagrammatic portrayal of the components of a semicircular canal is shown in Fig. 11.1. Each canal consists of a fluid filled tube, both ends of which join in a bulge in the tube referred to as the ampulla. Inside the ampulla is a brush of hairs which touches the top of the ampulla and is called the cupula. Movements of the cupula are registered by sensory nerve cells which pass the information back to the brain along the vestibular nerve.

A description of the mechanics of a semicircular canal was originally derived by van Egmond, Groen and Jongkees (1949), but the presentation given here follows the more recent analyses of Milsum (1966) and Wilson and Melvill Jones (1979). The mechanics are simplified by considering the canal to be a closed fluid - filled tube in which the cupula acts like a hinged flap. The simplified canal can be described by the equation describing a second order linear system.

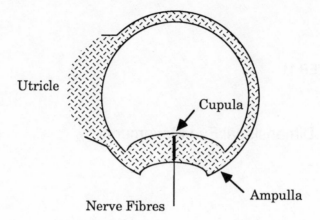

Utricle

Cupula

Ampulla

Nerve Fibres

FIG. 11.1. Schematic diagram of the components of a semicircular canal. The utricle is a sac to which the canal is connected.

When the skull is moved the resulting flow of the canal fluid must be such that the force due to the inertia of the fluid balances the forces due to the viscous drag of the fluid moving round the canal and to the stiffness of the cupula spring. Let ψ specify the angular position of the skull and θ specify the angular position of the canal fluid, as shown in Fig. 11.2, then the equation describing the system is:

$$J\frac{d\theta^2}{dt^2} = b(\frac{d\psi}{dt} - \frac{d\theta}{dt}) + k(\psi - \theta)$$

where

J = moment of inertia of the canal fluid
b = viscous force per unit angular velocity of fluid with respect to the canal
k = spring force per unit angular displacement of fluid with respect to the canal

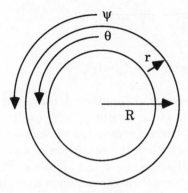

FIG. 11.2. Variables used in the analysis of the mechanics of a semicircular canal. ψ is the angular position of the skull and θ is the angular position of the canal fluid. R is the radius of the semicircular canal and r is the radius of the canal tube.

Let the displacement of the fluid with respect to the canal be denoted by $\phi = \psi - \theta$, then the equation of the system can be rewritten as:

$$J\frac{d\psi^2}{dt^2} = J\frac{d\phi^2}{dt^2} + b\frac{d\phi}{dt} + k\phi$$

If the input to the system is taken to be the acceleration of the head, then the corresponding transfer function is:

$$T(s) = \frac{\dfrac{J}{k}}{(\dfrac{J}{k})s^2 + (\dfrac{b}{k})s + 1}$$

and in the case of the semicircular canals, the second order system is formed by two first order systems in series so that the denominator of this transfer function can be expressed as a product of two factors:

$$T(s) = \frac{T_1 T_2}{(T_1 s + 1)(T_2 s + 1)}$$

where $T_1 T_2 = J/k$ and $T_1 + T_2 = b/k$.

van Egmond, Groen and Jongkees determined the time constant T_1 by rotating subjects at a constant velocity until there was no sensation of movement, and then stopping the movement suddenly and asking the subject to report when the sensation of movement stopped. Since the input to the canal system is the acceleration of the head rotation, stopping a constant rotation corresponds to an impulse function and so has a response which is the difference of two exponentials, an example of which was shown in Fig. 10.5. The decay of the response is dominated by the long time constant, and van Egmond, Groen and Jongkees found that the decay of sensation of movement could be fitted with an exponential curve with a time constant of 10 seconds.

Since the long time constant T_1 is very much greater than the short time constant T_2 it follows from the relationships between the time constants that $T_1 \approx b/k$ and $T_2 \, b/k \approx J/k$. So $T_2 \approx J/b$. An estimate of this time constant can be made indirectly from calculated values of J and b.

Any rotating body can be thought of as being a collection of infinitely small particles of mass dm, and it follows that the moment of inertia of the body is given by the integral over the whole body of the moments of inertia of each of the particles. The moment of inertia of a particle of mass dm located at a distance R from the axis of rotation is given by the product $R^2 dm$, and so the moment of inertia J of a rotating tube is given by:

$$J = \int_{volume} R^2 dm$$

The mass of the canal fluid is given by the product of the volume of the fluid in the narrow bore tube, the utricle and the ampulla with the density r of the canal fluid. Curthoys, Markham and Curthoys (1971) estimated from anatomical measurements that the volume of fluid in the canal is 4.9485 mm^3. Let the radius of the semicircular canal be R, as shown in Fig. 11.2, then the moment of inertia is given by:

$$J = 4.9485 \ \rho R^2$$

The density of the canal fluid is approximately 0.001 gm per mm^3 so:

$$J = 0.0388 \ \text{gm mm}^2$$

The viscous moment b can be obtained by applying Poiseuille's law[1], which relates the quantity of fluid Q flowing through a tube with radius r and of length l to the pressure p per unit area at the end of the tube by the formula :

---

[1] The derivation of the law is based upon the assumption that during smooth flow of fluid through the tube, the layer of fluid touching the tube is stationary, the layer next to the stationary layer is just moving and so on to the layer at the centre of the tube, which is moving fastest. Let the velocity at a distance x from the centre be v, then the velocity gradient is dv/dx and the viscous force per unit area is η dv/dx, where η is the coefficient of viscosity.

The force due to the pressure p per unit area applied at the end of the tube, is balanced by the viscous drag of the fluid moving along the length l of the tube so:

$$p\pi x^2 = - \eta \frac{dv}{dx} 2\pi x l$$

which can be rearranged to give the equation

$$- x dx = (\frac{2\eta l}{p}) dv$$

At the wall of the tube x = r and v = 0 so integrating between x = r and x = x gives:

$$\int_r^x x dx = \int_0^v \frac{2\eta l}{p} dv$$

Evaluation of these integrals leads to an expression for the velocity at a distance x from the centre of the tube:

$$v = \frac{p}{4\eta l}(r^2 - x^2)$$

Let dq be the volume flowing between radii x and dx, then:

$$dq = 2\pi x dx. v = \frac{p\pi x}{2\eta l}(r^2 - x^2) \ dx$$

therefore

$$Q = \int_0^r \frac{p\pi x}{2\eta l}(r^2 - x^2) \ dx = \frac{p\pi r^4}{8\eta l}$$

$$Q = \frac{p\pi r^4}{8\eta l}$$

Curthoys, Markham and Curthoys obtained average values of r = 0.163 mm and R = 2.8 mm from measurements of the bone which contains the canals.

In the case of a semicircular canal the length of the tube is equal to the circumference of the circle along the centre of the tube, so $l = 2\pi r$. Poiseuille's equation can be rearranged and the value for l substituted to give a formula for p:

$$p = \frac{16\eta RQ}{r^4}$$

Hence the overall viscous force f associated with movement of a volume of fluid Q through a tube with a cross - sectional area of πr^2 is:

$$F = \frac{16\eta\pi RQ}{r^2}$$

If the angular velocity of the fluid is one radian per second then:

$$Q = \pi r^2 R$$

and so

$$F = 16\eta\pi R^2$$

hence the viscous moment per unit angular velocity is:

$$b = 16\eta\pi^2 R^3$$

and since a quarter of the canal is taken up by the wider utricle, the effective viscous moment is:

$$b = 12\eta\pi^2 R^3$$

A typical value for h is 0.001 mm/gm/sec so b = 2.6 gm/mm per sec. Hence T_2 = 0.0388 / 2.6= 1 / 67.01 secs.

The Neural Integrator

The VESTIBULO - OCULAR REFLEX acts to keep the gaze direction aligned with the target and so ensures a stable retinal image despite head movements. If the head moves in one direction, the reflex produces a compensatory eye movement which is in the opposite direction to the head movement but of the same size.

Jones and Milsum (1965) used the Bode plot of the canal system to show that the canals effectively signal head velocity. The range of frequencies associated with naturally occurring head movements lies between 0.1 to 5 cycles per degree. Within this range the semicircular canals integrate the acceleration of the head , so that the deflection of the cupula is proportional to head velocity. The Bode plot for the canal is shown in Fig. 11.3. Integration of a sinusoidal function of angular frequency w reduces the amplitude of the function by 1/w, and when plotted on a logarithmic scale against frequency, this quantity lies on a straight line, as shown in Fig.11.3a. Similarly, since integration of a sine wave converts it into a cosine wave and vice versa, an integrator produces a ninety degree phase change at all frequencies, as reflected in the phase plot of the canal.

From the definition of the Laplace transform it follows that the transform of the differentiation operation is s, so the transform of head acceleration is equal to the transform of head velocity multiplied by s. Using this substitution, the transfer function of the canal system with head velocity as the input is equal to:

$$T(s) = \frac{T_1 T_2 s}{(T_1 s + 1)(T_2 s + 1)}$$

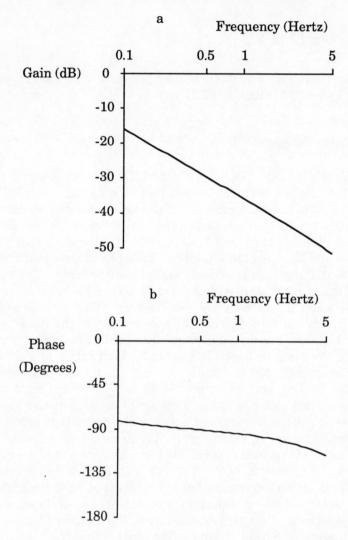

FIG.11.3 Bode diagram of the canal system. a) Gain plot b) Phase plot.

At the low head velocities associated with naturally occurring head movements $T_2w \ll 1$ and so the transform can be approximated by a first order system:

$$T(s) = \frac{T_1 T_2 s}{T_1 s + 1}$$

Buettner, Büttner and Henn (1978) recorded the responses of neurons in the vestibular nuclei of monkeys to sinusoidal head rotations in the dark. They found that the gain and phase changes of the responses with respect to head velocity could be modelled by a first order system with a time constant in the range 10 to 25 seconds, depending on the monkey. However, when the animals were sedated during the recordings, the time constants that fitted the results were in the range 4 to 7 seconds. These neurophysiological results show that the long time constant of the canal is approximately 4, rather than 10 seconds. The persistence of the subjective sensation of movement is only obtained after a neural mechanism has boosted the responses of the nerve fibres from the canals to low frequency head movements.

One of the advantages of studying the simpler vestibular system, as opposed to the visuomotor system, is that the neural operations are easier to isolate. If an eye is pulled round and then released, then it returns to its original resting position, so the eye muscles need a position signal if the eye is to be held in place. Robinson (1968) pointed out that it follows from the mechanics of the canals and eye muscles that for the eye to be held in its final position once a head movement stops, there must be a NEURAL INTEGRATOR which converts the velocity signal to a position signal. Subsequent work by Robinson and his co - workers has revealed that the neural integrator has been incorporated into the control of fast eye movements, so that changes in gaze direction are also specified in terms of a velocity signal.

Saccadic Eye Movements

Van Gisbergen, Robinson and Gielen (1981) recorded from burst neurons in monkeys. These neurons are located in the reticular formation close to the abducens nucleus and fire an average of 12 milliseconds before the begining of the saccade. Their main finding was that the firing of the burst cells was a function of MOTOR ERROR, which is defined to be the difference between the actual eye position and the target eye position. When the firing patterns of a burst cell associated with different sized saccades were plotted against motor error, then it was found that the patterns superimposed. The average of these patterns was described by a function of motor error e of the form:

$$f(e) = \begin{cases} 1100(1 - \exp(- \frac{e+c}{10})) & \text{if } e > -c \\ 0 & \text{otherwise} \end{cases}$$

A plot of the function with the offset term c set to zero is shown in shown in Fig.11.4.

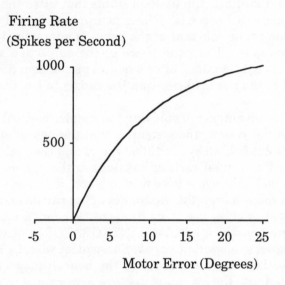

FIG. 11.4. Firing pattern of burst cells.

Van Gisbergen, Robinson and Gielen devised a model in which a nonlinear function of the motor error, as given by the difference between the the target gaze direction g* and the actual gaze direction g, is computed by the burst cells and this signal is passed directly to the eye muscles to provide a pulse of innervation to move the eye fast. In addition, the signal from the burst cells is integrated to provide the step change in innervation necessary to hold the eye in place. A simplified block diagram of the model is shown in Fig. 11.5; in the actual model separate pathways were used for the agonistic and antagonistic muscles.

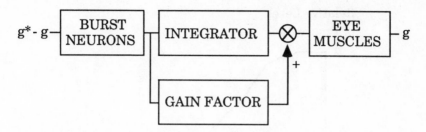

FIG.11.5. Integrator model for the generation of saccades.

The model for the eye muscle plant was based on recordings from oculomotor neurons. Typically, a motoneuron increases its firing as its associated muscle contracts, responding in direct proportion to a linear combination of the position, velocity and acceleration of the eye. During slow eye movements the firing pattern of a motoneuron can be approximated by the second order function:

$$f(g) = kg + r\frac{dg}{dt} + m\frac{d^2g}{dt^2}$$

This firing pattern reflects the signal needed to drive a second order system. The mechanical system of the extraocular muscles can be modelled by two first order systems in series, one of which has a time constant of r/k and one of which has a time constant of m/r. In their model Van Gisbergen , Robinson and Gielen used values of 0.15 and 0.004 seconds for the time constants.

The motoneuron firing patterns recorded during saccades show a characteristic burst of activity followed by a change in their tonic level of activity and the model predicts this characteristic pulse - step pattern of innervation. The pulse of innervation is required to produce the fast movement of the eye and the step change in innervation is needed to hold the eye in its new gaze direction. Fig. 11.6 shows the innervation signal delivered to the eye muscles, according to the model, during a 20 degree saccade. Following Van Gisbergen, Robinson and Gielen the gain factor was set to a value of 0.15, to produce the appropriate time course for the saccade.

Relative Level
of Innervation

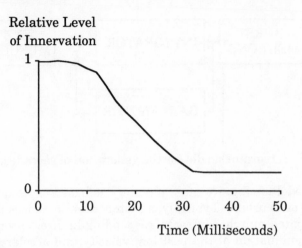

Time (Milliseconds)

FIG.11.6. Plot of the predicted time course of the innervation to the eye during a 20 degree saccade. There is an initial burst of innervation followed by a steady state change in innervation which holds the eye in its new resting position.

If saccade duration is plotted against amplitude, then a steadily increasing curve is obtained, and if peak velocity is plotted against amplitude than a curve which levels off is obtained.   These characteristic relationships between saccade amplitude, duration and peak velocity have been termed the MAIN SEQUENCE by Bahill, Clark and Stark (1975), and have proved to be very useful in identifying the action of the saccadic mechanism, For instance, the quick phase of nystagmus has a similar main sequence to that of saccadic eye movements and so it can be inferred that the same neural mechanism is involved in the generation of both types of eye movement.   A detailed example of this approach can be found in the investigation of congenital nystagmus carried out by Abadi and Worfolk (1989).

The characteristic plot of peak velocity against amplitude for a monkey shown in Fig. 11.7, was predicted by the integrator model. The computed curves match the experimental findings and so provide evidence for the validity of the model, and the success of the model suggests that even an approach as simple as averaging the responses of different neurons can be an effective strategy for unravelling their functional role.

Peak Velocity

(Degrees per Second)

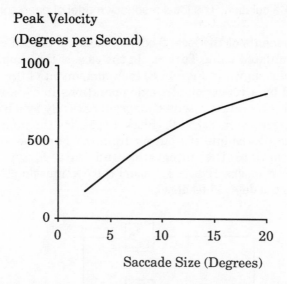

Saccade Size (Degrees)

FIG. 11.7. Characteristic plot of peak velocity against saccade size for a monkey, predicted by the gaze control model.

The model developed by Van Gisbergen, Robinson and Gielen was actually more comprehensive, in that signal for current eye position g was provided by a feedback loop within the model. In the LOCAL FEEDBACK MODEL the motor error is computed by subtracting a signal specifying eye position which is taken from the output of the integrator, as shown in Fig. 11.8. A delay of 5 milliseconds was included in the feedback path to take into account the lag in the movement of the muscle plant, when estimating the actual gaze angle.

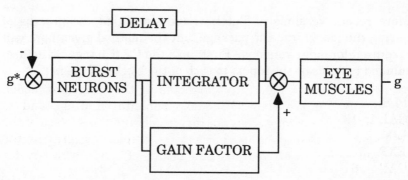

FIG.11.8. Simplified version of the local feedback model of saccadic gaze control.

Example Calculation: The local feedback model of gaze control

The components of the local feedback model of saccadic gaze control can be simulated using Tutsim. In the case of the simplified version of the model shown in Fig. 11.8, each component of the model can be simulated by a collection of single operations in Tutsim. If each of these operations is represented diagrammatically by a block, then the model appears as in Fig.11.9. Block 1 specifies the input g*, blocks 2 through to 6 calculate the output from the burst neurons, blocks 7 and 9 simulate the integrator and gain factor components respectively, blocks 10 and 11 model the eye muscle plant and block 12 models the delayed feedback.

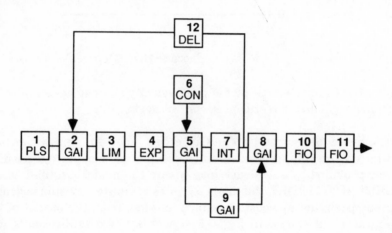

FIG. 11.9. Block diagram of the Tutsim implementation of the local feedback model shown in Fig.11.8.

More recent versions of Tutsim have simplified the process of entering the model into the package, but the method given here will be required for older versions. First , use the CS (Change Structure) command to describe the inputs to each of the blocks. Type in

1, PLS
2, GAI, 1, -12
3, LIM, 2
4, EXP, -3
5, GAI, -4, 6
6, CON
7, INT, 5

8, GAI, 7, 9
9, GAI, 5
10, FIO
11, FIO
12, DEL

followed by a carriage return.   Next, use the CP(Change Parameters) command to specify the parameters associated with each of the blocks. Type in:

1, 0, 0.1, 20
2, 0.1
3, 0, 100000
5, 1100
6, 1
7, 0
8, 1
9, 0.15
10, 1, 0.15, 0
11, 1, 0.004, 0
12, 0.001, 0.005, 0

again followed by return. To plot the position of the eye, which corresponds to the output from block 11, use the CB (Change plotBlocks) command. The first entry in the CB command specifies the timescale on the horizontal axis. Type in:

0, 0, 0.1
11, 0, 25

followed by return. Finally, specify the time units of the simulation using the CT (Change Time) command. Type in:

0.001, 0.1

The model is now ready to run. Type in SD (Start simulation: results to Display), and a plot of the time course of a twenty degrees saccade will appear on the screen. It easy to change the parameters of the blocks, to appreciate how the model works. For instance, to change the maximum firing rate of the burst neurons from 1100 to 800, as might occur with a nerve palsy, type in CP, followed by:

5, 800

The model now predicts a slower saccade. The outputs of the normal model and the altered model are plotted together in Fig. 11.10, for comparison.

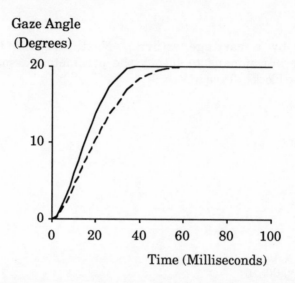

FIG. 11.10. Outputs from the model of the normal system (solid line) and a system in which the maximum firing rate of the burst neurons has been reduced (broken line), resulting in a slower saccade.

Summary

The response of the semicircular canals corresponds to a second order system with time constants of 10 and 1/67 seconds.

The semicircular canals signal head velocity, so that their output has to be integrated neurally to obtain the position signal needed to hold the eyes in their final gaze position.

The neural integrator is also used in saccadic eye movements to convert the signal from the burst neurons into a position signal.

CHAPTER 12

Three - Dimensional Eye Movements

The analysis given in chapter 6 revealed that the retinal disparities associated with stimuli restricted to the horizontal plane are qualitatively different from those associated with three - dimensional objects. Purely horizontal disparities can always have arisen from viewing a real object, but this is no longer true when both horizontal and vertical disparities are allowed. A similar situation arises in the context of eye movements, in that analysis of the control of three - dimensional eye movements shows that the task is qualitatively different from the control of one - dimensional eye movements.

The Three Dimensional Vestibulo - Ocular Reflex

The simplest component of the vestibulo - ocular reflex lies in the path which directly transforms the head velocity signal into an eye velocity signal, and the three - dimensional nature of this path was analysed by Robinson (1982), using a matrix formulation. Let h be a vector which specifies the angular velocity of the head, then the velocity signals of the canals can be calculated by multiplying h by the canal matrix C, which specifies the orientations of the canals. Similarly, let e be a vector which specifies the angular velocity of the eye, and M be a matrix which specifies the axes of rotation of the muscles, then multiplication of the neural signal to the muscles by M gives the eye velocity e. It follows that a matrix equation for the whole pathway takes the form:

$$e = MNC\, h$$

where N is a matrix which describes the neural transformation of the velocity signal.

There are two sets of semicircular canals, symmetrically placed about the midline. Each set contains a horizontal, anterior and posterior canal. The anterior canal makes an angle of around 40 degrees with the midline and the posterior canal makes an angle of around 125 degrees with the midline. The six semicircular canals can be grouped in pairs, according to their planes. The angle between the anterior and posterior semicircular canals is approximately 90 degrees so that the left anterior canal is aligned with the right posterior canal and similarly the right anterior canal is aligned with the left posterior canal

The orientations of the planes of the semicircular canals have been determined by Blanks, Curthoys and Markham (1975). The experimental technique involves surgically exposing the semicircular canals and then measuring the positions of a number of points along each canal with a probe attached to a micromanipulator. The canal matrix is built up by writing the orientation vector of the pair of horizontal canals into the first row, the orientation vector of the right - anterior / left - posterior pair into the second row and the orientation vector of the remaining pair into the third row. Using a right handed system of Cartesian base vectors, the resulting matrix has the values:

$$
C = \begin{bmatrix} 0.0 & 0.927 & -0.374 \\ 0.674 & 0.155 & 0.722 \\ -0.674 & 0.155 & 0.722 \end{bmatrix}
$$

Rotation of an eye is produced by six extraocular muscles, which are also grouped in three pairs: the lateral and medial rectus muscles, the superior and inferior rectus muscles and the superior and inferior oblique muscles. The positions of the extraocular muscles when both eyes are directed straight ahead are shown in Fig. 12.1. The recti muscles have their origin at the back of the orbit, as does the superior oblique, whilst the inferior oblique arises at the front of the orbit on the nasal side. The lateral and medial recti, referred to as the horizontal recti, lie on either side of the eye and the superior and inferior recti, referred to as the vertical recti, lie above and below the eye respectively. The superior oblique passes through a loop of cartilage at the front of the orbit and back over the upper

portion of the eye, attaching to the eye underneath the superior
rectus. The inferior oblique passes under the eye, outside the inferior
rectus and attaches to the eye underneath the lateral rectus.

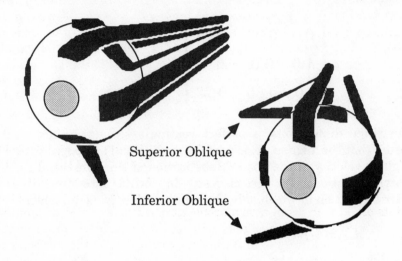

Superior Oblique

Inferior Oblique

FIG. 12.1. Positions of the extraocular muscles with the eyes looking
straight ahead. The recti muscles attach to the front of the eye,
whereas the obliques attach to the back of the eye.

Surprisingly, the axes of rotation of the muscles can be assumed to
be fixed with respect to the orbit, because of the broad insertions of the
muscles, which are approximately 10 millimetres wide.   The
significance of the wide insertions of the muscles was first pointed out
by Helmholtz (1910), who used the superior rectus as an example.
When the eye is pointing straight ahead, the effective point of
insertion of the muscle is assumed to lie at the midpoint of the
insertion of the muscle. When the gaze is directed nasally it is mainly
the temporal fibres of the superior rectus that are stretched and so
the effective point of insertion moves temporally. When the gaze is
directed temporally the opposite occurs, in that it is mainly the nasal
fibres that are stretched and so the effective point of insertion moves
nasally. Hence the effective axis of rotation of the superior rectus
remains approximately constant, irrespective of gaze direction. For
the vertical recti, the plane of the muscles makes an angle of 23
degrees with the midline, and for the obliques the angle is 51 degrees.
The matrix of the axes of rotation of the muscles is formed by writing
the orientation vector of the muscle plane of the horizontal recti into
the first column, the orientation vector of the muscle plane of the

vertical recti into the second column, and the orientation vector of the muscle plane of the obliques into the third column. Using a right handed system of base vectors again, the matrix M for the right eye is equal to:

$$M = \begin{bmatrix} 0.0 & 0.92 & -0.63 \\ 1.0 & 0.0 & 0.0 \\ 0.0 & 0.36 & 0.78 \end{bmatrix}$$

In three dimensions, a perfect vestibulo - ocular reflex would ensure that the angular velocity of the eye is equal and opposite to the angular velocity of the head. Substitution of this constraint in the matrix equation for a perfect vestibulo - ocular integrator gives a matrix equation in which only the neural matrix N is unknown:

$$U = MNC$$

where U is the matrix:

$$U = \begin{bmatrix} -1 & 0 & 0 \\ 0 & -1 & 0 \\ 0 & 0 & -1 \end{bmatrix}$$

This matrix equation can be solved numerically to give N :

$$N = M^{-1} U C^{-1} = \begin{bmatrix} -0.99 & -0.25 & -0.26 \\ 0.14 & -1.04 & 0.19 \\ 0.21 & -0.34 & -0.9 \end{bmatrix}$$

Example Calculation: The neural matrix for a cat

Measurements of the orientations of the semicircular canals in cats were made by Blanks, Curthoys and Markham (1972). Type the components of the canal matrix into a spreadsheet in Wingz, select the cells containing the matrix and a destination cell, and then choose inverse from the menu, to obtain the inverse of the canal matrix.

Canal Matrix C			Inverse of Canal Matrix C^{-1}		
0.00	0.93	-0.37	0.00	0.72	-0.72
0.69	0.34	0.64	0.89	0.26	0.26
-0.69	0.34	0.64	-0.47	0.65	0.65

The origins and insertions of the extraocular muscles in the cat were measured by Ezure and Graf (1984). Repeating the steps used with the canal matrix gives the inverse of the muscle matrix:

Muscle Matrix$M$			Inverse of Muscle Matrix M^{-1}		
0.06	0.87	-0.54	0.00	1.00	-0.11
0.97	0.05	0.09	0.85	0.08	0.54
-0.24	0.48	0.83	-0.49	0.24	0.86

As in the example given in chapter 4, one can use the matrix multiply option from the menu to calculate the successive matrix products required to calculate the neural matrix. Begin by typing in the elements of the matrix U :

-1.00	0.00	0.00
0.00	-1.00	0.00
0.00	0.00	-1.00

Select U first, C^{-1} next, a destination cell last and then choose multiply from the menu to obtain the matrix UC^{-1}:

-0.00	-0.72	0.72
-0.89	-0.26	-0.26
0.47	-0.65	-0.65

Finally, repeat the multiplication operation with M^{-1} and $UC^{-1}$to obtain the neural matrix N:

-0.94	-0.19	-0.19
0.18	-0.98	0.24
0.19	-0.27	-0.97

The implication of the neural matrix is that there are three main connections, corresponding to the elements n_{11}, n_{22} and n_{33}, each of which links one canal pair to one muscle pair. This result is in keeping with the physiological findings of Szentágothai (1950), who stimulated single semicircular canals in cats and dogs. He surgically exposed a semicircular canal and then inserted a fine tube filled with saline into the canal. The canal could then be stimulated by raising or lowering the pressure in the saline. He also removed the eyes of the animals, so that the resulting length changes of the stretched muscles could be recorded. He found that stimulation of the horizontal canal led to contraction of the ipsilateral medial rectus and the contralateral lateral rectus. Stimulation of the anterior canal led to contraction of the ipsilateral superior rectus and the contralateral inferior oblique. Finally, stimulation of the posterior canal led to contraction of the ipsilateral superior oblique and the contralateral inferior rectus.

Euler Angles

The component of the vestibulo - ocular reflex which converts the velocity signal into position signal is more complicated in three dimensions because the end result of a sequence of rotations depends on the order in which they are carried out. This component of the reflex can be analysed by using matrices to describe the individual rotations, so that the overall rotation can be expressed as a matrix product.

The geometry of a rotation is shown in Fig.12.2 where a pair of Cartesian base vectors e_1 and e_2 are rotated through an angle a into the new pair of Cartesian base vectors e_1' and e_2'.

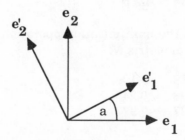

FIG. 12.2. Rotation of base vectors

The new set of base vectors can be expressed in terms of linear combinations of the original set of base vectors:

$$e_1' = \cos a \; e_1 + \sin a \; e_2$$

$$e_2' = - \sin a \; e_1 + \cos a \; e_2$$

Hence the ROTATION MATRIX associated with the transformation is equal to:

$$R = \begin{bmatrix} \cos \theta & \sin \theta \\ -\sin \theta & \cos \theta \end{bmatrix}$$

In three dimensions, the rotation matrix which describes a clockwise rotation of the base vectors through an angle a around the e_3 direction is:

$$R_3 = \begin{bmatrix} \cos \theta & \sin \theta & 0 \\ -\sin \theta & \cos \theta & 0 \\ 0 & 0 & 1 \end{bmatrix}$$

Similarly, the appropriate rotation matrices for clockwise rotation around the e_1 and e_2 axes are:

$$R_1 = \begin{bmatrix} 1 & 0 & 0 \\ 0 & \cos \theta & \sin \theta \\ 0 & -\sin \theta & \cos \theta \end{bmatrix}$$

and

$$R_2 = \begin{bmatrix} \cos\theta & 0 & -\sin\theta \\ 0 & 1 & 0 \\ \sin\theta & 0 & \cos\theta \end{bmatrix}$$

If A is a matrix which describes one set of Cartesian base vectors in terms of another, then each of the rows of A must be orthogonal since they represent orthogonal unit vectors. In matrix terms, the orthogonality of the rows implies that:

$$A^T A = \begin{bmatrix} 1 & 0 & 0 \\ 0 & 1 & 0 \\ 0 & 0 & 1 \end{bmatrix}$$

Any square matrix which satisfies this equation is referred to as an ORTHOGONAL MATRIX. By definition of an orthogonal matrix it holds that $A^{-1} = A^T$. The only transformations which satisfy the definition of orthogonality are reflections and rotations.

An appropriate system of coordinates for describing rotation of a rigid body about a centre of rotation O is provided by a specification of a line through O and a rotation of the eye around that line. This system requires three angles, referred to as EULER ANGLES. The first two angles specify the orientation of the line and the third specifies the rotation of the body about that line. In the context of movements of the eyes the most important visual direction is specified by the line, referred to as the LINE OF FIXATION, which passes through the centre of the fovea and the centre of rotation of the eye. Euler angles can be used to specify the orientation of the line of fixation and the rotation of the eye about that line.

The angles are defined by a sequence of rotations which transforms one set of Cartesian base vectors into another. One of the sets (e_1, e_2, e_3) is fixed in space and the other (e_1', e_2', e_3') is fixed with respect to the body. Fig. 12.3 shows the two sets of Cartesian base vectors in relation to the eye. The set e_1, e_2, e_3 is fixed with respect to the head and the set e_1', e_2', e_3' is fixed with respect to the eye. The head based system of axes is orientated so that the e_3 direction lies along the PRIMARY POSITION of the line of fixation, which is the position which the eyes adopt when an observer fixates a point straightahead on the horizon with the head erect. For convenience the e_1 base vector is set to lie in a horizontal plane and the e_2 base vector is set to lie in a vertical plane. When the eye is in the primary position the two sets of base vectors are coincident.

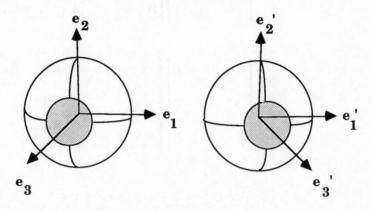

FIG. 12.3. Head and eye fixed systems of base vectors.

The first two Euler angles (ϕ, θ) specify the e_3' direction with respect to the fixed set of base vectors, and the third angle (ψ) specifies the rotation of the body about the e_3' direction. The angle ϕ is given by the clockwise rotation about e_3 needed to rotate the plane spanned by the e_2, e_3 base vectors into the plane spanned by the e_3 and e_3' base vectors. The angle θ is determined by the clockwise rotation about the new e_1 direction which aligns e_3 with e_3'. Finally, the angle ψ specifies the clockwise rotation about the e_3' direction.

For Euler's system of orientation angles, let

$s_\phi = \sin \phi$
$c_\phi = \cos \phi$
$s_\theta = \sin \theta$
$c_\theta = \cos \theta$
$s_\psi = \sin \psi$
$c_\psi = \cos \psi$

then

$$E \ (\phi, \theta, \psi) = R_3 \ (\psi)R_1 \ (\theta)R_3 \ (\phi)$$

$$= \begin{bmatrix} c_\psi & s_\psi & 0 \\ -s_\psi & c_\psi & 0 \\ 0 & 0 & 1 \end{bmatrix} \begin{bmatrix} 1 & 0 & 0 \\ 0 & c_\theta & s_\theta \\ 0 & -s_\theta & c_\theta \end{bmatrix} \begin{bmatrix} c_\phi & s_\phi & 0 \\ -s_\phi & c_\phi & 0 \\ 0 & 0 & 1 \end{bmatrix}$$

$$= \begin{bmatrix} c_\psi & s_\psi & 0 \\ -s_\psi & c_\psi & 0 \\ 0 & 0 & 1 \end{bmatrix} \begin{bmatrix} c_\phi & s_\phi & 0 \\ -s_\phi c_\theta & c_\phi c_\theta & s_\theta \\ s_\phi s_\theta & -c_\phi s_\theta & c_\theta \end{bmatrix}$$

$$= \begin{bmatrix} c_\phi c_\psi - s_\phi c_\theta s_\psi & s_\phi c_\psi + c_\phi c_\theta s_\psi & s_\theta s_\psi \\ -c_\phi s_\psi - s_\phi c_\theta c_\psi & -s_\phi s_\psi + c_\phi c_\theta c_\psi & s_\theta c_\psi \\ s_\phi s_\theta & -c_\phi s_\theta & c_\theta \end{bmatrix}$$

An infinitesimal rotatation ds of a rigid body, where s is a vector specifying the axis of rotation, can be expressed in terms of infinitesimal changes in the Euler angles ($\delta\phi$, $\delta\theta$, $\delta\psi$). The rotation of the eye from (ϕ, θ, ψ) to ($\phi + \Delta\phi$, $\theta + \Delta\theta$, $\psi + \Delta\psi$) is equivalent to the rotation that results from applying the infinitesimal rotations $\delta\phi e_3$, $\delta\theta e_1^*$ and $\delta\psi e_3'$, where e_1^* is the new direction of e_1 obtained after the rotation through ϕ. Because the rotations are infinitesimally small, the order in which they are carried out does not matter , and one has that:

$$\delta s = \delta\phi e_3 + \delta\theta e_1^* + \delta\psi e_3'$$

By expressing the vectors e_3 and e_1^* in terms of the e_1, e_2 and e_3 system of base vectors, one can obtain an expression for the infinitesimal rotation of the eye in terms of the head based system of base vectors:

$$\delta s = \delta s_1 e_1 + \delta s_2 e_2 + \delta s_3 e_3$$

One can use the matrix E to express e_3' in terms of the base vectors e_1, e_2 and e_3, and $e_1{}^*$ can be expressed in terms of e_1, e_2 and e_3 by applying the rotation matrix corresponding to the Euler angle f, so

$$\delta\theta e_1{}^* = \delta\theta \cos \phi \; e_1 + \delta\theta \sin \phi \; e_3$$

and

$$\delta\psi e_3' = \delta\psi \sin \phi \sin \theta \; e_1 - \delta\psi \cos \phi \sin \theta \; e_2$$
$$+ \delta\psi \cos \phi \; e_3$$

Substituting for e_3 and $e_1{}^*$ in the equation for an infinitesimal rotation gives the matrix equation:

$$\begin{bmatrix} \delta s_1 \\ \delta s_2 \\ \delta s_3 \end{bmatrix} = \begin{bmatrix} 0 & \cos\phi & \sin\phi\sin\theta \\ 0 & \sin\phi & -\cos\phi\sin\theta \\ 1 & 0 & -\cos\theta \end{bmatrix} \begin{bmatrix} \delta\phi \\ \delta\theta \\ \delta\psi \end{bmatrix}$$

Tweed and Vilis (1987) pointed out that descriptions of three dimensional rotations, of which Euler angles are an example, have implications for the mechanism of the vestibulo - ocular reflex. When only rotations about one axis are considered, ϕ and ψ are both zero and the matrix equation simplifies to:

$$\delta s_1 = \delta\theta$$

and integrating both sides of this equation, it follows that the integral of the velocity signal gives the angle of rotation θ. However, this approach does not work in three dimensions. An example which Tweed and Vilis analysed involved a subject lying at an angle of 30 degrees to the ground and being rotated about an axis perpendicular to the ground, while fixating a target in the direction of the axis of rotation. In this situation the only rotation that the eye needs to make in order to maintain fixation is a torsional rotation about the line of fixation. If the subject rotates at 1 degree per second, then the angular velocity vector in head based coordinates is:

$$\delta s = \begin{bmatrix} 0 \\ \dfrac{\sin(30)}{57.3} \\ \dfrac{\cos(30)}{57.3} \end{bmatrix}$$

If δs_1, δs_2 and δs_3 are each integrated independently then the horizontal position of the eye predicted by the integral of δs_2 will continue to increase, so the calculated movement will not maintain fixation. If the matrix formulation for the instantaneous rate of change of the Euler angles is applied to this example, then the initial conditions are that $\phi = 0$, $\theta = 30°$ and $\psi = 0$, so the matrix equation is:

$$\begin{bmatrix} 0 \\ \dfrac{\sin(30)}{57.3} \\ \dfrac{\cos(30)}{57.3} \end{bmatrix} = \begin{bmatrix} 0 & 1 & 0 \\ 0 & 0 & -\sin(30) \\ 1 & 0 & -\cos(30) \end{bmatrix} \begin{bmatrix} \delta\phi \\ \delta\theta \\ \delta\psi \end{bmatrix}$$

and this equation is only satisfied if $\delta\phi = \delta\theta = 0$ and $\delta\psi = -1/57.3$, which is precisely the torsional rotation of the eye required to maintain fixation.

The angular velocity signal can still be converted to a position signal by solving the matrix equation for $\delta\phi$, $\delta\theta$ and $\delta\psi$ and then integrating each of these individually to obtain the orientation angles ϕ, θ and ψ. But Tweed and Vilis made the additional point that this is not possible without a position feedback loop as ϕ, θ and ψ are required for the calculation of $\delta\phi$, $\delta\theta$ and $\delta\psi$.

Orientation of the Eye

The next question to consider is what modifications to the model of saccade generation based on the neural integrator need to be made to extend it to three dimensions. Before considering changes in the direction of fixation, one has to define how the eye is orientated in three dimensions when a target is being fixated. The simplest expectation is that the orientation of the eye is determined by the mechanical system which supports it. For example in the Fick system shown in Fig. 12.4a, the eye is first rotated around a vertical axis through an angle of longitude θ and then rotated around an axis in the horizontal plane through an angle of latitude ϕ. In the Helmholtz sequence, the eye is first rotated around an horizontal axis through an angle of elevation λ and then rotated around an axis perpendicular to the plane containing the lines of fixation of the two eyes, through an angle of azimuth μ. A mechanical system which embodies Helmholtz's system of orientation angles is shown in Fig. 12.4b.

One way of appreciating the constraint imposed by the mechanical system is to imagine a torch being rotated according to these two systems. If the front of the torch is covered by a cardboard mask with a cross cut in it, then the projections of the cross on a plane surface facing the torch are as shown in Figs. 12.4c and 12.4d. With the Fick system shown in Fig. 12.4c, the vertical arm of the cross always remains vertical, and with the Helmholtz system shown in Fig. 12.4d, the horizontal arm of the cross always remains horizontal.

The orientation of the eye was initially investigated by using afterimages, which have a fixed location on the retina and so move with the eye, like the torch with the mechanical systems. Typically, the subject was given the afterimage of a cross in the primary position and reported on the apparent shape of the cross on a tangent screen in other gaze directions. The uniform finding was that the cross was distorted when gaze was directed along oblique meridians, as shown in Fig. 12.5. However, the most important conclusion from this study was that the apparent location of the cross was the same everytime that the gaze was directed at a particular point of fixation, no matter what location it had been directed at before. This discovery was summarised in DONDER'S LAW 'The orientation of the eye depends only on the final direction of the line of fixation.'

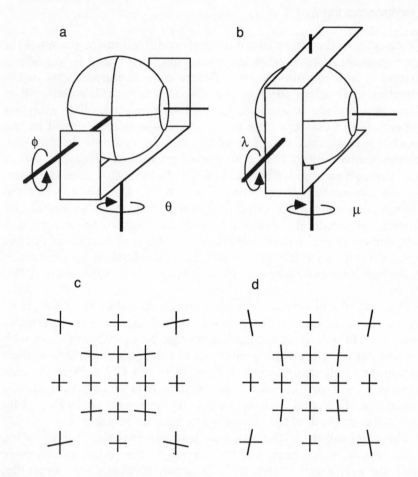

FIG. 12.4. Mechanical systems for describing the orientation of the eye. a) The Fick system. b) The Helmholtz system, c) Projection of a cross moved in accordance with Fick's system, d) Projection of a cross moved in accordance with Helmoltz's system.

Donder's law means that although the eye could rotate with three degrees of freedom, since it could rotate around the e_1, e_2 or e_3 directions, it effectively only rotates with two degrees of freedom. So what are the axes around which normal eye rotations occur? If an afterimage of an oblique cross was moved to a point of fixation along the associated oblique meridian, it was found that the shape of the cross did not change,so that the axis of rotation had to be perpendicular to the oblique meridian. This finding is summarised by

LISTING'S LAW which states that if the eye moves about a centre O so that the line of fixation moves away from the primary position OA to another position OB, then the displacement of the eyeball is equivalent to rotating it around an axis perpendicular to the plane AOB.

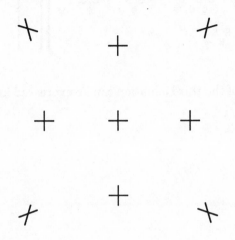

FIG. 12.5. Orientation of an afterimage of a cross

What distinguishes Listing's system of rotation from other systems such as that of Fick and Helmholtz is that it is the way of moving the eye which minimises the rotation of the eye around its line of fixation. Because of this, the relation between retinal directions and head fixed directions are least affected by movements of the eyes.

Specification of the Motor Error

Listing's law requires that for rotations away from the primary position, the axis of rotation must lie in the e_1e_2 plane. Since the axis of rotation is unchanged under the rotation, if the column matrix V specifies the coordinates of the axis of rotation then:

$$V = E^T(\phi, \theta, \psi)V$$

Helmholtz (1910) derived the constraint on Listing's system of orientation angles due to Listing's law by substituting the values $V = (v_1, v_2, 0)$ into this equation. Expanding out the elements of the

matrix gives the equation:

$$
\begin{bmatrix} v_1 \\ v_2 \\ 0 \end{bmatrix} = \begin{bmatrix} c_\phi c_\psi - s_\phi c_\theta s_\psi & -(c_\phi s_\psi + s_\phi c_\theta c_\psi) \\ s_\phi c_\psi + c_\phi c_\theta s_\psi & -s_\phi s_\psi + c_\phi c_\theta c_\psi \\ s_\theta s_\psi & s_\theta c_\psi \end{bmatrix} \begin{bmatrix} v_1 \\ v_2 \end{bmatrix}
$$

The solutions of the third equation can be expressed in the form:

$$v_1 = tc_\psi$$

and

$$v_2 = - ts_\psi$$

where t is a scalar constant. Substituting these values for v_1 and v_2 in the first row of the matrix equation gives:

$$tc_\psi = tc_\phi c_\psi^2 - ts_\phi c_\theta s_\psi c_\psi + tc_\phi s_\psi^2 + ts_\phi c_\theta s_\psi c_\psi$$

which simplifies to $c_\psi = c_\phi$. Similarly, substitution of the values for v_1 and v_2 in the second row of the matrix equation gives:

$$-ts_\psi = ts_\phi c_\psi^2 + tc_\phi c_\theta s_\psi c_\psi + ts_\phi s_\psi^2 - tc_\phi c_\theta s_\psi c_\psi$$

which simplifies to $-s_\psi = s_\phi$. These two constraints are satisfied when $\psi = -\phi$.

When Listing's law is obeyed then an infinitesimal rotation of the eye ds is described by the matrix equation:

$$\begin{bmatrix} \delta s_1 \\ \delta s_2 \\ \delta s_3 \end{bmatrix} = \begin{bmatrix} \cos\phi & -\sin\phi\sin\theta \\ \sin\phi & \cos\phi\sin\theta \\ 0 & 1+\cos\theta \end{bmatrix} \begin{bmatrix} \delta\theta \\ \delta\phi \end{bmatrix}$$

The same procedure as that used to derive the matrix equation describing an infinitesimal rotation in head based coordinates can be used to express the infinitesimal axis of rotation in terms of eye based coordinates. When the constraint implied by Listing's law is applied to the corresponding matrix equation:

$$\begin{bmatrix} \delta s_1' \\ \delta s_2' \\ \delta s_3' \end{bmatrix} = \begin{bmatrix} \cos\phi & -\sin\phi\sin\theta \\ \sin\phi & \cos\phi\sin\theta \\ 0 & \cos\theta-1 \end{bmatrix} \begin{bmatrix} \delta\theta \\ \delta\phi \end{bmatrix}$$

Comparison of the terms in these two matrix equations shows that:

$$\begin{bmatrix} \delta s_1 \\ \delta s_2 \\ \delta s_3 \end{bmatrix} = \begin{bmatrix} \delta s_1' \\ \delta s_2' \\ -\delta s_3' \end{bmatrix}$$

so that the axis of rotation must lie in the plane which bisects the e_1e_2 and $e_1'e_2'$ planes. This result shows that Listing's law also places a constraint on the location of the axis of rotation when the eye moves from a position away from the primary direction of gaze. The nature of this constraint is that if the line of fixation makes an angle w with the primary direction of the line of fixation, and is rotated about a fixed axis in accordance with Listing's law, then the axis of rotation must make an angle w/2 with the e_1e_2 plane, as shown in Fig. 12.6.

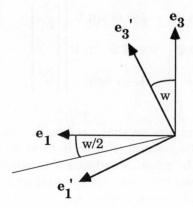

Figure 12.6. Axis of rotation for eye movements away from the primary position.

These results were first proved by Helmholtz (1910), who went on to introduce the term ATROPIC LINE for the normal to the plane in which the axes of rotation must lie. For any given direction of the line of fixation, the atropic line will lie in the same meridian as the line of fixation, but at half the angle of eccentricity. If the eye rotates about a fixed axis from its current position (ϕ,θ) to a target position (ϕ^*,θ^*) in accordance with Listing's law, then the fixed axis must lie in both of the planes of the axes of rotations associated with the two positions of the eyes. Hence the axis is given by the intersection of the two planes. Let the atropic line for the initial line of fixation be t and for the target position be t *, then a vector d in the direction of the required axis of rotation is given by the vector product of t and t *:

$$d = t_{\wedge} t *$$

Tweed and Vilis (1990) have demonstrated experimentally that Listing's law is obeyed during saccadic eye movements, so that when a movement is made then the rotation occurs about a fixed axis. Furthermore, this axis lies away from the e_1e_2 plane with half the angle of the line of fixation, as predicted. The implication of this finding is that the motor error E in three dimensions is not simply the difference between the target and actual gaze directions (E = g - g*), but also involves a specifiction of the axis of rotation which is in accordance with Listing's law (E = $t \wedge t$ *).

The descriptions of the vestibulo - ocular reflex and saccadic eye movements are still incomplete, in that the nature of binocular eye movements remains to be specified. Listing's law is only strictly true for distant targets, when the lines of fixation of the two eyes are parallel. When the eyes converge, it might be expected that the eyes would move according to the Helmholtz system of orientation, because the disparities are straightforward to interpret with this system of movement, as shown in chapter 6. Certainly, torsional movements of the eyes occur with convergence, but this is a long way from saying that the eyes move according to Helmholtz's system, and if the horizontal meridians of the two eyes do not remain coincident, then the nervous system will have to separate out the rotational components of the disparities, as well as the radial components, if the horizontal component which signals depth is to be isolated.

Example Calculation: Pattern of disparities with torsional eye movements.

The image p' in the coordinate system of the left eye of a point p, specified in a coordinate system fixed with respect to the head, and with its origin located at the midpoint between the two eyes, is given by:

$$p' = E^{T}(\phi_L, \theta_L, \psi_L)(p - \frac{s}{2})$$

where s is a vector equal to the interocular separation and ϕ_L, θ_L and ψ_L are the Euler angles which specify the orientation of the left eye. Similarly, the image p'' in the right eye is given by the equation:

$$p'' = E^{T}(\phi_R, \theta_R, \psi_R)(p + \frac{s}{2})$$

Let the interocular separation equal 65 millimetres and let the point of fixation be located 573 millimetres from the observer in the straight ahead direction, as shown in Fig. 12.7. As the point of fixation is in the horizontal plane $\phi_L = \phi_R = 90$ degrees, and $\theta_L = -\theta_R =$ Arctan (32.5/573) = 3.25 degrees. In this example it will be assumed that a differential cyclotorsion of one degree exists between the two eyes, as occurs during head tilt, so $\psi_L = \phi_L + 0.5$ degrees and $\psi_R = \phi_R - 0.5$ degrees.

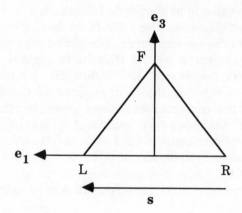

FIGURE 12.7 Viewpoint geometry.

In this example, the foregoing analysis will be used to extend the range of viewing geometries for which disparity field plots can be produced, using Mathematica. Begin by loading the Rotations.m and PlotField.m routines from the Geometry and Graphics packages respectively. The paths to these files will depend on the system that you are using to run Mathematica.

```
<<Rotations.m
<<PlotField.m
```

Next define a list of lists to hold the computed vector field:

```
temp = Table[i j k,{i,49},{j,2}, {k,2}]
```

where i, j and k must all be separated by spaces. The vector field is computed by the following set of commands. The first two lines compute the position of the point a frontal plane which passes through the point of fixation. The next four lines compute the images of the point in the left and right eyes respectively. In the next three lines the retinal disparity is calculated and stored.

```
Do[Do[x = Tan[(i-4)*5/57.3]*573;
    y = Tan[(j-4)*5/57.3]*573;
    a = {x - 32.5, y, 573};
    c = Rotate3D[a, -90.5/57.3, 3.25/57.3, 90.0/57.3];
    b = {x + 32.5, y, 573};
```

d = Rotate3D[b, -89.5/57.3,-3.25/57.3, 90.0/57.3];
h = ((c[[1]]/c[[3]]) - (d[[1]]/d[[3]]))*4000;
v = ((c[[2]]/c[[3]]) - (d[[2]]/d[[3]]))*4000;
temp[[i+(j-1)*7]] = {{x,y},{h,v}},
{i,7}],
{j,7}]

Finally the vector field is plotted with the command:

ListPlotVectorField[temp]

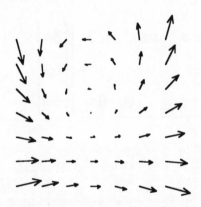

The first disparity field calculated in the example in chapter 6 gives the pattern of disparities associated with points on the frontal plane when no cyclotorsion is present.

Summary

Let (e$_1$, e$_2$, e$_3$) and (e$_1$', e$_2$', e$_3$') be two sets of right - handed Cartesian base vectors, fixed with respect to the head and eye respectively, then the orientation of the eye can be described by the Euler angles ϕ, θ, and ψ. The orientation angles ϕ and θ specify the meridian and eccentricity of the line of fixation, respectively. The orientation angle ψ specifies a rotation about the line of fixation. The matrix E which describes the rotation which transforms the head based system of base vectors into the eye based system of base vectors is:

$$
E = \begin{bmatrix}
c_\phi c_\psi - s_\phi c_\theta s_\psi & s_\phi c_\psi + c_\phi c_\theta s_\psi & s_\theta s_\psi \\
-c_\phi s_\psi - s_\phi c_\theta c_\psi & -s_\phi s_\psi + c_\phi c_\theta c_\psi & s_\theta c_\psi \\
s_\phi s_\theta & -c_\phi s_\theta & c_\theta
\end{bmatrix}
$$

An instantaneous change in the orientation of the eye, described by a vector δs , in head based coordinates, is related to the instantaneous change in the orientation angles by the matrix equation:

$$
\begin{bmatrix} \delta s_1 \\ \delta s_2 \\ \delta s_3 \end{bmatrix} = \begin{bmatrix} 0 & \cos\phi & \sin\phi\sin\theta \\ 0 & \sin\phi & -\cos\phi\sin\theta \\ 1 & 0 & -\cos\theta \end{bmatrix} \begin{bmatrix} \delta\phi \\ \delta\theta \\ \delta\psi \end{bmatrix}
$$

This equation implies that the Euler angles ϕ, θ, and ψ have to be supplied to the mechanism which converts the angular velocity of the eye to changes in the Euler angles. The rate of change of each of the Euler angles can then be integrated to give a position signal. Hence, the velocity to position integrator of the vestibulo - ocular reflex and saccadic eye movement controller, has to be replaced in three dimensions by a velocity to position converter, which requires a position feedback signal.

The orientation of the line of fixation is described by Listing's law which entails that $\psi = -\phi$. During saccadic eye movements, the eye rotates around a fixed axis in accordance with Listing's law, so that in three dimensions the motor error signal supplied to the saccadic eye movement controller must also specify the axis of the rotation, as well as its size.

CHAPTER 13

Conclusion

Obviously, it would be interesting to pursue the transformations of the physical stimulus through the visual system to the point where one could describe the conscious image, which is what one actually sees, but our subjective worlds are built on properties of the optical, neural and motor images which remain elusive. Consider the apparent stability of the visual world - although one's eyes are constantly moving around, one does not notice this movement. Rather one has the impression of a stable visual world, with the appearance of objects being unaffected by the movements of their images over the retina.

The direction of a retinal image can only be interpreted with the addition of information concerning the position of the eyes within the head, and one possibility is that this information is supplied by sensory receptors in the extraocular muscles. Another possibility is that, accompanying each movement of the eyes, a copy of the motor signal is sent to the perception centres, and the position of each object is formed by combining the motor signal with the retinal signal. This copy of the motor signal was referred to as the COROLLARY DISCHARGE by Sperry (1950).

A phenomenon which was introduced early on into the discussion about the mechanism involved in the stability of the visual world is that of the apparent movement of the visual world that occurs when the eye is nudged with a finger. If one pushes upwards then the objects in the field of view appear to move downwards. Helmholtz (1910) deduced that the apparent position of objects is not judged on the basis of information supplied by sensory receptors in the eye muscles, since any such mechanism would register mechanical disturbance of the eye.

The obvious explanation of the eyepress phenomenon is that the finger rotates the eye, so that the line of fixation moves upwards and the images on the retina of stationary objects move upwards, so that the objects appear to move downwards, taking into account the inversion of the retinal image. Stark and Bridgeman (1983) pointed out that the assumption that the direction of the line of fixation changes when the eye is pressed is incorrect. They demonstrated that fixation is maintained during eyepress, by showing that subjects do not lose the high resolution associated with the fovea. As eyepress can cause astigmatism, they chose a colour discrimination task rather than a spatial resolution task. The subjects could successfully discriminate the colour of a 6 minute by 6 minute of arc square, which was either red or green. Since this task is only possible with foveal vision, the subjects must have been maintaining fixation.

In fact the eyepress results in a translation of the eye in the orbit, with a minimal change in gaze angle. Rather the eye maintains fixation, but the motor signals to the muscles which are necessary to maintain fixation have to be changed. The corollary discharge associated with the new motor signals is not matched by any change in the retinal signal, so apparent motion of the visual world is seen. The century long misinterpretation of the eyepress phenomenon illustrates the difficulty of relating the optical, neural and motor images to each other.

References

Abadi, R.V., and Worfolk, R. (1989) Retinal slip velocities in congenital nystagmus. *Vision Research*, 29, 195 - 205.

Bahill, A.T., Clark, M.R. and Stark, L.R. (1975) The main sequence, a tool for studying human eye movements. *Mathematical Biosciences* , 24, 191 - 204.

Blakemore, C. and Campbell, F.W. (1969) On the existence of neurones in the human visual system selectively sensitive to the orientation and size of retinal images. *Journal of Physiology (London)*, 203, 237 - 260.

Blanks, R.H.I., Curthoys, I.S. and Markham, C.H. (1972) Planar relationships of semicircular canals in the cat. *American Journal of Physiology*, 223, 55 - 62.

Blanks, R.H.I., Curthoys, I.S. and Markham, C.H. (1975) Planar relationships of the semicircular canals in man. *Acta Oto - Laryngolica* , 80, 185 - 196.

Bowmaker, J.K, Dartnall, H.J.A., Lythgoe, J.N. and Mollon, J.D. (1978) The visual pigments of rods and cones in the rhesus monkey, *Macaca Mulatta* . *Journal of Physiology (London)*, 274, 329 - 348.

Buchsbaum, G. and Gottschalk, A. (1983) Trichromacy, opponent colour coding and optimum colour information transmission in the retina. *Proceedings of the Royal Society of London. Series B* , 220, 89 - 113

Buettner, U.W., Büttner, U. and Henn, V. (1978) Transfer characteristics of neurons in vestibular nuclei of the alert monkey. *Journal of Neurophysiology* , 41, 1614 - 1628.

Campbell, F.W. and Robson, J.G. Application of Fourier analysis to the visibility of gratings. *Journal of Physiology (London)*, 197, 551 - 566.

Curthoys, I.S., Markham, C.H. and Curthoys, E.J. (1977) Semicircular duct and ampulla dimensions in cat, guinea pig and man. *Journal of Morphology*, 151, 17 -34.

Egmond, A.A.J. van, Groen, J.J. and Jongkees, L.B.W. (1949) The mechanics of the semicircular canals. *Journal of Physiology (London)*, 110, 1 - 17.

Enroth - Cugell, C. and Robson, J.G. (1966) The contrast sensitivity of the retinal ganglion cells of the cat. *Journal of Physiology (London)*, 187, 517 - 552.

Ezure K. and Graf. W. (1984) A quantitative analysis of the spatial organisation of the vestibulo-ocular reflexes in lateral- and frontal- eyed animals - I. Orientation of semicircular canals and extraocular muscles. *Neuroscience*, 12, 85 - 93.

Hawken, M.J. and Parker, A.J. (1987) Spatial properties of neurons in the monkey striate cortex. *Proceedings of the Royal Society of London. Series B*, 231, 251 - 288.

Helmholtz, H. von (1910) *Treatise on Physiological Optics*. Translated by J.P.C.Southall, 1924, New York: Dover.

Hering, E. (1879) *Spatial Sense and Movement of the Eye*. Translated by C.A. Radde, 1942, Baltimore: American Academy of Optometry.

Hertz, J., Krogh, A and Palmer R.G. (1991) *Introduction to the Theory of Neural Computation*. Massachusetts: Addison - Wesley Publishing Company.

Hubel, D.H. (1988) *Eye, Brain and Vision*. New York: W.H. Freeman and Company.

Hubel, D.H. and Wiesel, T.N. (1962) Receptive fields, binocular interaction and functional architecture in the cat's visual cortex. *Journal of Physiology (London)*, 160, 106 - 154.

Ingling, C.R. and Martinez - Uriegas, E. (1983) The relationship between spectral sensitivity and spatial sensitivity for the primate r-g X-channel. *Vision Research*, 12, 1495 - 1500.

Jones, G.M. and Milsum, J.H. (1965) Spatial and dynamic aspects of visual fixation. *IEEE Transactions on Bio-Medical Engineering*, 12, 54 - 62.

Le Grand, Y. (1945) *Physiological Optics*. Translated and updated by S.G. El Hage, 1980, Berlin: Springer.

Longuet-Higgins, H.C. (1982) Appendix to paper by John Mayhew entitled: "The interpretation of stereo-disparity information: the computation of surface orientation and depth". *Perception*, 11, 405-407.

Longuet-Higgins, H.C. and Prazdny, K. (1980) The interpretation of a moving retinal image. *Proceedings of the Royal Society of London. Series B*, 208, 385-397.

Mayhew, J. (1982) The interpretation of stereo-disparity information: the computation of surface orientation and depth. *Perception*, 11, 387-403.

Mayhew, J.E.W and Longuet - Higgins, H.C. (1982) A computational model of binocular depth perception. *Nature*, 297, 376 - 378.

Milsum, J.H. (1966) *Biological Control Systems Analysis*. New York: McGraw - Hill Book Company.

Ogle, K.N. (1936) The correction of aniseikonia with ophthalmic lenses. *Journal of the Optical Society of America*, 26, 323-337.

Ogle, K.N. (1950) *Researches in Binocular Vision*. New York: Hafner

Publishing Company, 1964.

Oja, E. (1982) A simplified neuron model as a principal component analyser. *Journal of Mathematical Biology* , 15, 267 - 273.

Robinson, D.A. (1968) Eye movement control in primates. *Science* , 161, 1219 - 1224.

Robinson, D.A. (1982) The use of matrices in analyzing the three - dimensional behaviour of the vestibulo - ocular reflex. *Biological Cybernetics* , 46, 53 - 66.

Sanger, T.D. (1989) Optimal unsupervised learning in a single - layer linear feedforward neural network. *Neural Networks* , 2, 459 - 473.

Smith, V.C. and Pokorny, J. (1975) Spectral sensitivity of the foveal cone photopigments between 400 and 500 nm. *Vision Research*, 15, 161 - 171.

Sperry, R.W. (1950) Neural basis of the spontaneous optokinetic response produced by visual inversion. *Journal of Comparative and Physiological Psychology* , 43, 482 - 489.

Stark, L. and Bridgeman, B. (1983) Role of corollary discharge in space constancy. *Perception & Psychophysics*, 34, 371 - 380.

Szentágothai, J. (1950) The elementary vestibulo - ocular reflex arc. *Journal of Neurophysiology* , 13, 395 - 407.

Tweed, D. and Vilis, T. (1983) Implications of rotational kinematics for the oculomotor system in three dimensions. *Journal of Neurophysiology* , 58, 832 - 849.

Tweed, D. and Vilis, T. (1990) Geometric relations of eye position and velocity vectors during saccades. *Vision Research* , 30, 111 - 127.

Vakkur, G.J. and Bishop, P.O. (1963) The schematic eye in the cat. *Vision Research*, 3, 357 - 381.

Vakkur, G.J., Bishop, P.O. and Kozak, W. (1963) Visual optics in the cat, including posterior nodal distance and retinal landmarks. *Vision Research*, 3, 89 - 324.

Van Gisbergen, J.A.M., Robinson, D.A. and Gielen, S. (1981) A quantitative analysis of generation of saccadic eye movements by burst neurons. *Journal of Neurophysiology* , 45, 417 - 442.

Vos, J.J. and Walraven, P.L. (1970) On the derivation of the foveal receptor primaries. *Vision Research* , 11, 799 - 818.

Wheatstone, C. (1838) On some remarkable, and hitherto unobserved phenomenon of binocular vision. *Philosophical Transactions of the Royal Society* , 128, 371 - 394. 2 Plates.

Wilson, V.J. and Melvill Jones, G. (1979) *Mammalian Vestibular Physiology*. New York: Plenum Press.

Wright, W.D. (1969) *The Measurement of Colour*. London: Hilger and Watts. 4th Edition.

Wysecki, G. and Stiles, W.S. (1967) *Color Science*. New York: John Wiley & Sons Inc.

APPENDIX

Software Packages

The software packages used in the example calculations are all commercially available. Wingz is a trademark of

Informix Software Inc.,
16011 College Boulevard,
Lenesca,
Kansas 66219, U.S.A.

Excel is a product of

Microsoft Corporation,
One Microsoft Way,
Redmond WA 98052 - 6399, U.S.A.

Mathematica is a registered trademark of

Wolfram Research Inc.,
100 Trade Center Drive,
Champaign,
IL 61820 - 7237, U.S.A.

European distribution is handled by

Wolfram Research Europe Ltd.,
Evenlode Court,
Main Road,

Long Hanborough,
Oxon OX8 2LA, U.K.

Tutsim is a product of

Meerman Automation,
P.O.Box 154,
7160 AC Neede,
The Netherlands

North American distribution is handled by:

Tutsim Products,
200 Californian Avenue,
Palo Alto,
California 94306

A number of other comparable software packages are already available, so one should not feel bound to use a package from this list. In practice the choice of which package to use is more a matter for individual preference. For instance, the calculation of the system matrix of the schematic eye of the cat given in chapter 4 can be done using either Excel or Mathematica rather than Wingz.

To use Excel to perform the calculation, type the elements of the refraction and translation matrices into the first two columns (A and B) of a worksheet, as shown:

	A	B	C	D
1	1.00000	-43.87398		
2	0.00000	1.00000		
3				
4	1.00000	0.00000	1.00000	-43.87398
5	0.00049	1.00000	0.00049	0.97850
6				
7	1.00000	5.06971	1.00248	-38.91326
8	0.00000	1.00000	0.00049	0.97850
9				
10	1.00000	0.00000	1.00248	-38.91326
11	0.00338	1.00000	0.00388	0.84697
12				
13	1.00000	-30.33333	0.88484	-64.60483
14	0.00000	1.00000	0.00388	0.84697
15				
16	1.00000	0.00000	0.88484	-64.60483
17	0.00547	1.00000	0.00872	0.49359
18				
19	1.00000	-27.13043	0.64830	-77.99604
20	0.00000	1.00000	0.00872	0.49359

The next two columns are used to hold the succeeeding product matrices. The first product matrix is calculated by typing into cell C4 the formula:

    = A4*A1 + B4*A2

and the into cells C5, D4 and D5 respectively, the formulae:

    = A5*A1 + B5*A2
    = A4*B1 + B4*B2
    = A5*B1 + B5*B2

The next product matrix is computed by typing in the formulae:

    = A7*C4 + B7*C5
    = A8*C4 + B8*C5
    = A7*D4 + B7*D5
    = A8*D4 + B8*D5

into cells C7, C8, D7, and D8 respectively. The formulae entered in cells C7-8 and D7-8 can be copied into cells C10-11 and D10-11, C13-14 and D13-14 and so on to the final product matrix which is held in cells C19-20 and D19-20.

With Mathematica, calculation of the intermediate product matrices can be skipped. The successive refraction and translation matrices are entered as lists of lists, (remembering that each entry is only evaluated when the enter key is pressed):

    a = {{1,-43.87398},{0,1}}
    b = {{1,0},{0.00049,1}}
    c = {{1,5.06971},{0,1}}
    d = {{1,0},{0.00338,1}}
    e = {{1,-30.33333},{0,1}}
    f = {{1,0},{0.00547,1}}
    g = {{1,-27.13043},{0,1}}

The system matrix is calculated by typing in:

    s = g.f.e.d.c.b.a

and the result can be displayed in the form of a matrix using the command:

    MatrixForm[s]

which will result in the system matrix being displayed:

    0.648304   -77.996
    0.00871847   0.493587

Index

In this index definitions are given in bold, e.g.: rotation matrix **173**; example calculations in italic, e.g.: quadrature filters *123-6*. An asterisk after the reference indicates the summary section at the end of the chapter, e.g.: learning rules 92*-3*.